# HYGGE

How to Hygge Without Buying Into the Hype

(Enjoy the Present Through the Healthy Danish
Art of Happiness)

**Patrick Howlett**

Published By Bella Frost

**Patrick Howlett**

All Rights Reserved

*Hygge: How to Hygge Without Buying Into the Hype (Enjoy the Present Through the Healthy Danish Art of Happiness)*

ISBN 978-1-77485-275-0

Legal & Disclaimer

The information contained in this book is not designed to replace or take the place of any form of medicine or professional medical advice. The information in this book has been provided for educational and entertainment purposes only.

The information contained in this book has been compiled from sources deemed reliable, and it is accurate to the best of the Author's knowledge; however, the Author cannot guarantee its accuracy and validity and cannot be held liable for any errors or omissions. Changes are periodically made to this book. You must consult your doctor or get professional medical advice before using any of the suggested remedies, techniques, or information in this book.

Upon using the information contained in this book, you agree to hold harmless the Author from and against any damages, costs, and expenses, including any legal fees potentially resulting from the application of any of the information provided by this guide. This disclaimer applies to any damages or injury caused by the use and application, whether directly or indirectly, of any advice or information presented, whether for breach of contract, tort, negligence, personal injury, criminal intent, or under any other cause of action.

You agree to accept all risks of using the information presented inside this book. You need to consult a professional medical practitioner in order to ensure you are both able and healthy enough to participate in this program.

# TABLE OF CONTENTS

# Introduction

Hygge is more than a passing fancy for Danes It's a logical process that is a key element of their ongoing success on world satisfaction diagrams and could be the answer to stress and anxiety of modern-day living.

A major disruption in the city of Copenhagen can do more than satisfy your desire for new experiences. It will satisfy your primary desire to feel more relaxed.

SAS will take passengers between Birmingham, Manchester, London Heathrow, Aberdeen and Edinburgh specifically to Copenhagen.

The best part about the hygge way of life can be that, in the main it's accessible to everyone. Since most of the hygge-related activities cost nothing, nobody should be deprived of trying these activities due to money.

But for many Americans the most important issue is time. Contrary to Denmark which is a place where people from all levels of society enjoy lots of time for relaxation in Americans are a different story. U.S. has a frantic society. Everyone seems to be engaged all the time - the richest significantly more than those who are poor. In reality, it's almost an act that we are proud Americans to boast over how busy we are, and the short time we have to take off as it makes us appear efficient and important.

This chaotic way of life is why hygge can be so useful to us. It forces us to take a step take a step back and relax to a point that isn't able to fall into place for many of us. The act of putting aside some time in our schedule for long walks as well as potluck dinners and pre-packaged game nights will allow us to get away from the rat race of work or acquiring and spending and just enjoy. Furthermore, if Denmark has any precedents it will be happy for it.

# Chapter 1: The Origins of Hygge and What It Can Mean

As mentioned in the introduction Hygge is an Danish term that refers to an expression of everyday togetherness. It's a state of comfort and warmth like the warmth that is experienced when drinking a glass of wine in the evening with a good friend. It is a noun that is a feeling, a social setting, and an act, however it is a verb that can be used in a reflexive way it can be used in the following manner "Let Us Hygge in a group." Hygge can also be an adjective, as in the instance, "A small Hyggeligt cottage in the woods." The other term that is akin to Hygge is uhyggelit. It can be translated as scary.

The term Hygge was not originally in it's Danish dialect, however it is came from Norwegian In simple terms it translates to "well-being". It was introduced across Denmark during the 18th century. It has been an integral aspect of Danish culture since then. It's simple to see the reason for this if we take a look at the harsh winters that are common in Denmark. They're brutally cold and the temperature dropping lower than zero are not uncommon in any way. There are the option of 17 hours in darkness during the day that can be a burden on anyone who is sane. There are only four months between spring and summer and autumn is almost not even a thing.

Many people who live in a more chilly climate know how crucial it is to have an inviting and warm environment. An open fireplace inside a mountain lodge or a bottle of Russian Vodka, a bowl of hot chicken soup and a rug made of bear skin can all be attributed to enhancing that warm feeling. Hygge encompasses all of these and more. Hygge doesn't need to be considered a winter phenomenon however, it is the season that marks its start. Hygge is a form of living. Hygge is dependent on each individual. In some instances it is possible for one person to be comfortable in a single-room apartment, while another might be suffocated and uncomfortable in such a tiny space.

The ideas behind Hygge can be broken down into a handful of key terms:

Atmosphere, especially with the proper lighting.

Presence - Think about clicking of the entire technology.

Pleasure - Cook clever and often unique food.

Egality - This is just "we are superior to me".

The concept of gratitude is to be grateful for all you have...Now.

Harmony - This isn't the place to indulge in egos and bragging.

Comfort - Being aware of your surroundings.

Truce - Not having any drama or conflicts.

It is the concept of bringing people closer

Shelter - Feeling of security.

Hygge is about self-care and being connected to others and creating a space which is safe and comfortable. It is believed that the Happiness Institute of Denmark have discovered that it could be Danes social connections that make them the most happy and that Hygge places small gatherings of friends in the center.

In the last 10 years there has been a bit of a worldwide revival in the Hygge lifestyle. It's unclear whether the generation of millennials has contributed to this trend or if people have only started to realize it is true that Danish are among the most happy people around the globe, even in the midst of difficult circumstances, or perhaps that's the story. The rebirth is focused on making the ordinary extraordinary by incorporating rituals into everyday things like making tea or dining at your home. It's about letting technology go for a time and adopting basic practices. Simple practices might include setting a fire, arranging flowers in a gorgeous vase or using your grandmother's china, which is typically stored in a closet somewhere.

Hygge is a great way to spend time with friends and family at all year round or simply as a person curling in a book. With heart conditions, hypertension and addiction to drugs so prevalent in our contemporary world, the simple act of Hygge is a method to put aside the stress for a time, take a look at our lives and shift toward a calmer life. This is the practice of having a brief break from all things and people that creates tension in our lives.

Your home could appear a bit different if you are a fan of this style. It is likely that you will decorate your home with more leather or wood. You may get an overall natural vibe to your home. It is possible to focus more on lighting based on the activities that take place in the space such as, for instance, less lighting in the dining area or soft light within the bedroom. The walls can get painted in order to give a more tranquil environment, and candles can be visible throughout the room.

To master practicing the practice of Hygge and incorporate it into our everyday lives it is important to realize that we're slowing down an instant and creating a moment. In the hospitality sector, they have benefited from this trend for a long time by giving guests an experience that is not only a bed and television. They are looking to surpass the expectations of their guests by inventing the amenities that they can provide to the space. It could be a fire pit that is set in the backyard, or a sports court, or an aromatherapy lotion on the nightstand. We live in a world that is fast-paced and Hygge is a reminder to slow down and take a breath each and every day. Hygge is a popular concept at the Morley College of London has even begun to teach Hygge as a method of teaching Hygge as part of their Danish Language course. It's not uncommon to listen to students discuss their future Hygge celebration regardless of whether it's eating out at a local restaurant or a class with gentle music. The Danish tradition is one of things that are low-cost and less expensive things. Maybe this is why they're thought to be the most happy people on earth. Maybe they've discovered the secret to a fulfilled life.

It is time to look at our schedules to see whether there are any activities we can eliminate to reduce the stress we feel in our lives. The question to consider is, do you think Susie really require an additional activity after school? Do you think that playing three or four games more crucial than spending time with Susie? These are questions we must be asking ourselves, and talking about in our homes with family members. When do we step off the active bandwagon and discover what really matters? Susie could be doing something that she dislikes because she believes Mom or Dad will want the task. The perception of reality is the basis for our actions, and an intimate conversation with our spouses, children and children could be just what the doctor recommended especially when the doctor is practicing this art form called Hygge.

Change isn't always easy however it is the reality of life. There is a saying that education or knowledge is the key ingredient that will alter the course of the world. Understanding the Hygge way of life can assist you in making the necessary changes in your everyday life - changes that bring happiness as well as an overall sense of wellbeing to your family. Westerners have lost sight of how important family is. This is due to the reality that children grow and graduate from college or get married, and half of them relocate away from their home and away from their immediate family. Young couples have only the time of their lives with their children, which is why it's crucial to take a step back and choose your activities carefully.

It is crucial to ensure that you create an enjoyable and happy one. It is important to create an area that people feel excited to visit and that your kids' friends would like to gather. There's no place as home and, hopefully, Hygge will be a excellent beginning.

The subsequent chapters of this book will aid you to begin your journey to a more comfortable and comfortable life. The ideas you'll discover are by no by any means the only suggestions or even "The Bible of Hygge" However, they are beneficial in their application and could provide you with an understanding of how to practice your life in Hygge.

## Chapter 2: The 12 Steps to Integrate into Your Life "Hygge" the secret to Danish Happiness

Denmark is the most happiest nation worldwide According to an annual report by The UN has been conducting since 2012. A lot of points, beyond the Scandinavian welfare system that the reason for happiness lies in the concept of hygge (pronounced something like Huu-gue but it's better to listen here) This concept does not have a simple definition and that is often written about.

Verne Mikkel Larsen stated, "It's hard to find any word that describes it. It would be a combination of the feeling of being welcomed, well-being, and having a place that makes you feel at ease at ease, relaxed and comfortable." Communication from The Danish Embassy to Madrid to him is about something social, having fun and sharing it with others. His colleagues Julie Thomsen and Deputy Consul Birte Stecher have a belief that peace, stress-free moments to take small steps that bring us joy, you can do it alone.

However, within the Scandinavian diplomats' representation, they don't think that hygge is related to bad weather as Quartz recently claimed but they do believe that winter and autumn are more vulnerable. Thomsen says, "It is more necessary because it's cold and dark".

Strategies to incorporate hygge in our life: Find the right timing.

The idea is to set aside time to doing things that make us feel content with those we love as well as with our own. "In Denmark, we think of spending our time productively, work and accomplish all of our daily chores. "On on top that they have time to care for themselves and unwind from the commitments, by doing "little items," the woman says.

Let your home be open.

Hygge can be found everywhere. A barbecue outside in summer and a stroll through the park, a bite or a meal in an eatery can be relaxing. However, Danes prefer to gather at home, and are not interested in those Spaniards that they might be in bars, or which is why they are more open.

Create an environment that is conducive to growth.

Be sure to take care of the lighting that is warm. Play good background music. A fireplace is a great option and candles are an essential part. A fresh bouquet of flowers placed on a table, and a clean tablecloth and even eating by yourself, they can add an individual touch that will lead to pure pleasure. It's about taking care of the small things to make you are comfortable.

Beware of anything that could disturb the state of rest.

It can be a transition from being peaceful to enjoying a moment at peace, and it's not a good idea to dwell on work, issues, stress of the day and hurriedness.

Television, tablets and phones also block the social networks that create Hygge.

It's best to use it in the small committee.

It's all about the dimension of your home and you However, as per what they have to say it's best to do it by utilizing smaller cores. Additionally, it makes sense since it's more relaxing to talk to one another rather than having several gatherings.

Imagine the menu.

In the winter and fall The Danes are not thinking of the night without hot beverage. Cooking for a group is also a common practice. It is possible to gather with their family or friends, and cook meatballs using the traditional recipe or bake cakes. They also love Grod, a sort of porridge, or porridge that recalls their childhood, since Hygge is also full of nostalgia. But, the best way to enjoy hygge is to be a good excuse to purchase some cheeses that are creamy and a bottle wine and enjoy it under the light of a candle.

Remember your ancestral ancestors.

There are those who believe that the concept of Hygge is a result of doing things that your ancestors might recognize. The Danes who we've consulted believe that it is associated with traditions and things or activities with sentimental significance. Sitting down to tea with the kitchen of your grandmother is Hygge, as per Larsen. For Stecher who has been living in Spain for over 40 years and is still a fan of Danish practices and customs, getting furnishings of her grandparents feels like breathing in the scent of his parents' home again and it's an extremely hygge-like feeling for her. Explore every day the classic Scandinavian advent calendar which cuts down days till Christmas as it transports them back to their childhoods when they were together with their parents.

Relax and enjoy yourself.

While hygge's main purpose is to do with pleasure more than it does with things or actions specifically, certain elements can help. For instance, candles. They provide warmth and light in a time as darkness and cold rule Scandinavia as well as comfortable clothes. According to Thomsen I like to stay in bed on Sundays with my duvet on longer than I normally do while reading a book and a cup of tea or coffee. Or, I like to curl in a sofa under blankets with hot warm tea and watch the latest film.

Do things that are hyggelig.

It is crucial to choose something you love and, typically it's something straightforward. Board games played with people from your family or with friends are enjoyable and hyggelig. Also, Christmas is a great time, but Easter (which is the hunt for chocolate eggs hidden in the bushes) is more enjoyable than hyggelig, according to Larsen. Some things are considered hygge to certain individuals, and not for all. For instance, Thomsen, with 24 years of age, thinks the idea that Pokemon playing with your friends can work, but not dependent on mobiles because it's about having quality time together. For Stecher all things that have to involve mobiles or video games is not relaxing and, consequently, is not a good idea.

Escape from places that don't fit with.

The synonym for this word is uhyggelig. However, this is more of the horror film, which is filled that is filled with blood, terror, and so on. What the Danes are referring to is everything that does not allow people to be at ease. For Larsen as an example, it's impossible to achieve the feeling of a relaxing atmosphere in the atmosphere of a Spanish bar that has seating made of plastic, shaded spaces, as well as fluorescent tube.

Express it.

In Denmark the country, it's an expression they use frequently, adds to the adjective, noun or adverb and verb. It is used to describe the comfy sweater that you put on, telling your kids "we will watch the latest movie and have a snack" or "we will have a game of Trivial with our friends and enjoy a relaxing time". It's often used to tell with your acquaintances how wonderful you feel in that moment and also to say goodbye to them after the meal that was extremely cozy.

Take note of the pleasure.

A meal or an extended Spanish desk with friends could be considered hygge however what distinguishes the Danes is the ability to recognize and identify that moment of happiness. They are aware of what's happening and are having fun, something that is similar to continuous awareness that is typical of the Nordic way. "It is very compatible when it comes to slow living and is similar to Buddhist," says Larsen. The goal for Stecher, "is to live in the moment, and to enjoy the moment."

What is the reason PEOPLE Are So Afraid of HYGGE?

It's more than just an excuse to stay in bed or renewal. It could also be a method to be more content in the dark and cold winter months and something that Denmark has a lot of experience with.

People are looking for all things that serotonin, a neurotransmitter, can do, including the human touch, friendship and even hugs, according to A. K. Pradeep Neuro markers and the creator of "The Brain that buys."

"The commercial brand name Peel Huge, and what makes it a serotonin booster," Dr. Pradeep versus CNBC Make It. In winter (high season to indulge in) everyone all over the world seek out activities that boost serotonin levels and lessen stress.

Wiking claims that comfort is an "survival method" for those living in Nordic countries in which winters can be long and it is extremely dark at 5 pm. 4:00 pm (However you can do it throughout the year. "It is suggested to bring lunch or an outdoor barbecue with your friends in your park".

A geophysicist who emigrated into Copenhagen out of to the United States named Alex Calvert Nine years ago said to CNBC Make It that he was initially concerned about how the dark winters and long nights could influence his mood.

"But truthfully walking through the streets, you'll see candles and fires in the windows that are lit up at night when people are in the attic, talking," he tells CNBC Make It. "Even during the winter's coldest days there's still an underlying warmth ".

Based on Dr. Avery, it could assist in the application of some Hyde's principles particularly socializing, to assist someone with the blues.

People tend to be withdrawn and this only increases the feelings of depression and makes people more lonely, says Dr. Avery. "It is essential to stay with people who have a similar type of depression." Avery adds, "it is important to be around others."

Hygge events are an opportunity to enjoy a small ritual for those who are looking to experience friendship and "the warmth of the human community," Dr. Pradeep.

Americans spend much of their time at the computer or in front of the television late at night, which could impact their sleep, according to the doctor. Avery.

Hygge is, on contrary, encourages the use of screens, such as reading books and playing games or just engaging in conversation with your friends. It will result in a positive effect on your health He adds.

The word"coziness" is an individual way of being in a relationship with someone else that is dependent on the person you're with as well as where you are and what you're doing. What you see as being coziness is different between people. Many people say they are able to enjoy their time on their own, however they usually have informal interactions with family and friends. If you're enjoying yourself, you will often take a drink and eat together. All in all, cozy is the manifestation of the everyday joys of living. It doesn't require numerous things to create a warm environment, e.g. only a couple of candles or an assortment of candy for Friday can be enough to make a impact.

The concept of coziness is a reflection of certain values that are more generalized in Danish social life e.g., Coziness is closely linked to perceptions of equality. In these times, the power imbalances, inequalities or differences shouldn't be too obvious. The importance of being cozy in Denmark could be linked to the Danish climate, in which cold dry, wet and dark months encourage socializing.

The word"coziness" implies an ideal, peaceful as well as secure because these words concentrate on physical state or being while Danish and Norwegian are focused on mental states.

The opposite of cozy is haunting and can be applied from mild discomfort to catastrophic events. The phrases (anything that isn't coziness) are frequently employed as an understatement to stop swearing.

The English printed as well as the online version of Collins English Dictionary named "hygge" as a dry word (after "Brexit") as a word in their list of terms that were most popular in the UK in the year 2016. The announcement came in the wake of an era of intense focus in the United Kingdom regarding the idea of and the publication of a set of books featuring the word"hygge" in the title. Collins defines the word as "a conceptthat originated in Denmark that focuses on creating comfortable and welcoming environments that encourage well-being" ("a idea that originated in Denmark that is focused on creating a welcoming and beautiful environment that promotes well-belng ".

"The Dutch phrase, "gezelligheid", has the same concept of coziness with regards to coziness and comfort. It is German, "Gemutlichkeit" means the quality of warmth, kindness and belonging. It is the Norwegian term "cozy" is used to refer to an experience in the warmth of intimacy, love and a sense of belonging.

While many people see coziness as a good thing however, it can be a bit exclusive and introverted. Very few people are comfortable in a relationship with someone they don't have a relationship with, and it may be difficult to enter the places where entertainment takes place.

Is coziness uniquely Danish? In reality there are people who enjoy it in different countries too however they do not necessarily see the same significance the way it is in Denmark. That is, it is the concept of coziness, which holds an important place in Denmark and is what Danes frequently use to explain to foreigners what it means to be Danish.

Hygiene is an activity that is social which can create communities that are present in daily life. Hygge is one of the ideas that have been made it into the Danish canon. It is a concept of gathering for a social gathering, food customs and traditions of the holiday season, Danish design, and music culture, reading books and watching EM with 92 people and attending the festival. Also hygiene is a huge quantity, which is why there are so many Danes are not aware of the typical features of Denmark and, more importantly, is a part of Danish culture.

Everyone is at ease through different methods, because their physical and psychological characteristics are a factor along with their health status, as well as other aspects. Because of this, the same mattress could be to be comfortable for some, but firm or soft for others for instance, to mention a situation where comfort is essential for the mattress to perform.

People who have found the key to Happiness

THE PEOPLE

While we think that the most crucial decoration are rooms, houses are the rooms, this is not true that the most important thing is the people who utilize the space. The residents of a house are the primary focus and you must ensure that they feel at ease in the space they live in.

The Danes have been consistently at the top of the list of world's most happy citizens for years. The year 2016 was no exception. were ranked first at the top of the World Happiness Index - The United Nation Published a ranking of the world's most happy people every year. What makes the citizens of Denmark so happy as well as what could we take from the Danish people? Denmark isn't a particularly vast country, and its frigid and rainy weather doesn't encourage its inhabitants to spend much time outside. The history of Denmark isn't too positive either, since the Danes have been defeated in every war they've participated over the course of decades. If we consider some of the most expensive tax rates anywhere in the world, it's difficult to understand what makes they are Danes are so content.

It's been discovered that many aspects affect the happiness of Danes and contribute to the general feeling of wellbeing. The health care system is of high significance in this regard. It's not just the feeling of security, but also the general happiness. The inhabitants of Denmark are also more comfortable and open in the past few times. Health and education is free along with high-paying jobs and other benefits keep the Danes from being worried about their future, allowing them more time to focus on personal and social development.

It is interesting to note that the University of Warwick scientists also verified that the people of Denmark have a higher level of happiness than other nations due to the fact that joy is a fact of their DNA. Other races that are related to Danes are happier than those that aren't as fortunate in their genetic connections to them. In addition the fact that the average Dane also has higher levels of serotonin, also known as the happiness hormone that is responsible for our happiness.

However certain experts consider they believe that what is known as the Danish method of happiness is totally different. Based on the research of Professor Kaare Christensen at the University of South Denmark, Danes aren't putting very exigencies in life This is why they are able to enjoy the smallest things in life and be content with the everyday things that happen to them. This unique method lets them focus on what is essential in the world even in the face of many hardships. There is a reason that a widely-used phrase within Denmark that reads

"Modest but great". Do you think that's the definition of hygge? Let's see.

In order to find a gorgeous design for our furniture it is important to consider the comfort, and especially if it gives us a sense of wellbeing. When you are purchasing an sofa, the primary thing you should consider is whether it's comfortable, just like the chair or mattress on our beds.

Find tranquil colors

If your home is decorated with vibrant colors, you will never rest. neutral colours are the most popular and which are more resistant to fade away from. Get away from intense oranges, turquoise, or deep purples that use white cream or light yellow. Also, consider pastel colors. Danes tend to prefer monochromatic spaces in order to create more harmony. You should also look for simplicity of your hygge decor Do not overcrowd your space with unnecessary items.

Be aware of the minute things.

If you don't have many furniture pieces within your home You can add details that bring peace to areas. Take inspiration from memories from your family, friends or travels and what feels good to you when you look at it. You can also make use of handmade or recycled objects that convey an interesting story. The details that make a home distinctive and unique.

Do not forget the beauty of the beauty of nature and the green.

A key element of every house is wood since it is able to transport you closer to the natural world. The same is true if you have plants in your home, therefore, do not neglect to include some greenery in your home. Wood in all of its varieties provides warmth. Mix different textures and you'll be delighted with the outcome.

Make sure that lighting is of the highest importance.

Within the Nordic countries, such as Denmark daylight hours are shorter than Spain This is the reason they have curtains that are thin to maximize the natural light. The fireplace is also an ideal since it can, aside from the heating function, it also has the ability to illuminate. Make use of it whenever you are able to switch out the light, put out candles, and create peaceful environments.

Learn To Enjoy Loneliness

It is one of the rules that govern this style of living. Additionally, it's that the Danes have it spelled out. Every person deserves their own space, their time of quiet to indulge in their passions such as reading a good book or drawing, or even watching a favorite show. Don't let go of the pleasures you only are able to appreciate.

Make your own private spaces free of the normal and work environment and let yourself be a bit more free. Make a space for crafts or music of the things you love most however, don't deprive yourself of enjoying your interests over relationships with others that are equally important, even though there is plenty of time to do every thing.

Do nothing and enjoy it

This could be the idea that's at the edge of this way of living. You must know how to maximize the time you don't have for yourself, like the extra hour of sleep at a quiet area of your home drinking the tea you like, watching a film or music while closed in your eyes or doing nothing. Put aside the phone or computer, whatever gadget and just enjoy the time you've got to offer yourself These are the essentials of living.

# Chapter 3: What to Adopt Hygge in The Workplace

## 1. Create your work area as your own

H

Ygge is associated with taking a charge from the world around you, and turning the spaces you live in into mini-sanctuaries that let us sink in them at any moment.

In this regard, Soderberg proposes that we make our workplaces more personalized, as it is possible by focusing on things that let us escape from the routine of our daily routine and make an effort to take pleasure in those moments that will make you smile and fill your heart with joy.

"Bringing images, clippings or a mug that you love from the home or a jolly comic is an amazing way to bring character to our workplace," she says. "Numerous workplaces are designed in a sensible and organized way, but for those who want to feel a bit comfort, it's helpful in adding the character."

## 2. Let the outdoors in you

Hygge doesn't only apply to the comforts of our homes inside It is also possible to create feelings of hygge when we go out on a long walk or rummaging around for ordinary fruit, and enjoying the air we breathe on our skin.

Soderberg emphasizes that having plants to look after will help you recreate the joy we feel from the outdoors, not to mention the fact that they can make a significant impact on the mood of your workplace.

"My closet was lacking on living, which is why I brought some plants to add some shine," she lets us know. "I was inspired by my interior planner Christina B. Kjeldsen, who proposes the collection of a few plants so that you can have a stunning green area to feast you eyes.

"I brought a small bright and inexpensive Oxalis as well as a small Cactus that has a beautiful purple flower. They don't need any care at all; nevertheless, they're beautiful and attractive. As I get to work and start dressing and applying my make-up, I usually offer the oxalis a bit of water. This is now a element of my routine prior to my show."

3. As much as you can from lunchtimes

Do not take your lunch break and sit at your desk Wrap yourself warm, go outside to grab some food, do some things accomplished and walk around, or grab a book and find a quiet place to read.

4. Change the lighting in your office

"I require great lighting when making my makeup, which is why the mirror in my closet has lights surrounding it. Also, I have a reading light on my table, which is where I be reading my book," clarifies Soderberg.

"To create a cozy and warm lighting it is important to add a few bulbs that are warm, and a little orange, light throughout the room, creating the illusion of pools of light, like little rooms of light where you can get soaked by your work.

"A ideal working light for the table should be located in a position where the shade covers the bulb so that the light reflects directly onto the table and the work surface on the table. It does not reflect directly onto your eyes. This isn't beneficial for focusing as a source of hygge."

If your workplace allows candles, consider investing in a good scent one.

"There is a lot of hygge and hygge-like vibes in flame lights and I've carried one to the auditorium so that I can use it when I sit down to make my presentation," says Soderberg.

"The light that it produces is a way to be aware of my being different from all others in a distinctive way. It's a way to let me know that now is the right time to been set to get my work done in a relaxing and comfortable manner."

5. Make sure you have extra layers on hand

The colder winter months are settling in and battles for the air conditioner get heated it's an excellent idea to keep a few cozy layers in your workplace. This could include the cashmere-colored jumper or a dazzling scarf or a pair of socks (ideal for rainy days when it will soak your shoes straight through) or a soft cape cardigan. It's the closest to a suitable speed into a blanket that is working.

6. Pause for a moment

Making a conscious effort to take a break for a few minutes regardless of whether it's to pour a cup of tea into your personal mug, is vital to creating a cozy workplace. Make sure you have a stash of your favorite teabags in your cabinet and be sure to make use of them regularly.

7. Do not be confined to one spot.

There's no need to be in your office during the day. Soderberg suggests being creative when it comes to your workspace, ensuring that you are able to move around during various activities.

She says: "The most hyggelig thing in my closet is the two couches at the corner of the room. They consistently allow me to relax and relax while I study content alone with no other than me, or when I practice lines and discussing the material along with one of my colleagues.

"If your workplace is spacious enough to accommodate a sofa an easy chair to devote your entire time to, it could be a great option as opposed to sitting in front of the dining table.

"It is often a good idea to make your workday more cozy to comprehend messages, write plans for the day or phone someone while sipping tea at the table."

8. Create an office playlist

The music you listen to can keep the environment from being overly harsh or peaceful, no matter if it's getting everyone in the office to be in agreement on a radio show or just putting on your earphones or listening to the soothing sounds of music, it is crucial to keeping you in a well-being.

Try to select songs that invoke sentiments of comfort and connection whenever you can. Some suggestions include Mumford and Sons' I Will Wait and Radiohead's Everything in Its Right Place and Touch the Sky by Julie Fowlis.

9. Make sure you are happy at work

Hygge is currently in our vocabulary, however it is worth adding another Danish phrase to your vocabulary Arbejdsglaede. Arbejde refers to work, while glade is a synonym for happiness, therefore arbejdsglaede means "satisfaction with work."

In Denmark and the other Scandinavian countries working isn't just an opportunity to earn money and they sincerely wish to achieve a certain satisfaction with their work and happiness, in addition.

This is possible through flexible working hours, extraordinary employee benefits or regular preparing (Danes are driven to study new things) or by managers who make less immediate demands (they prefer laborers because they feel more empowered).

In any event, if you don't have this in your workplace it is possible to locate your arbejdsglaede through praising others around you, doing random acts of kindness in the workplace and by taking a regular amount of time off for yourself every day, and having natural products in the workplace to eat snacks throughout the duration of the day.

10. Connect with your coworkers

"Hygge is the sensation of being seen and felt as well as being in a natural environment that is popular," says Soderberg - that's why forming relationships with your colleagues is important. It doesn't matter if you're bringing everyone tea, getting an update on the day's events, holding individual feedback sessions for your clients, or even introducing unusual meeting places (try walking and talking, or even take everyone outside to hold up).

You can also plan an enjoyable event for all of you to try together, like going to a cafe in the area in the afternoon or having a drink on the patio after work.

"Snatch one of your brews after work, and let the covers fall and then hygge," proposes Soderberg.

In any case, your fun does not have to be limited to work You can also work out a sweepstakes, take an hour to play an evening game with your friends and try meditation sessions in the afternoon, or sit together for a relaxing meeting over a hot drink and some biscuits.

You can even create an enjoyable food rota and let people take their food to the market to buy handmade cakes or soup for work.

Whichever you pick is a good idea to dive in regardless of the outcome. there's nothing more cozy than making some time for others.

3 Ways that You can Implement the Principles of Hygge at the Workplace

There is a way to increase the feeling of comfort and satisfaction that is often associated to Hygge. In the workplace, this means creating a positive culture and offering a wide range of benefits, and ensuring that employees enjoy tiny moments of happiness and fulfillment as an integral element of their workday. Three ways to draw inspiration from Hygge and change the way you conduct your business.

1. Facilitate communication throughout the company

When it's done correctly, hygge at work should make everyone feeling energized and happy. It isn't possible in the absence of a strict top-down hierarchy with little communication between different posts. Instead, it's better to establish a formal system where every employee is considered an individual, and as a important contributor to business success.

Through opening up lines of effective communication within the workplace across the senior leadership, special department heads, officials and their assistants - and actively promoting the ideas of everyone in the workforce it is possible to create an environment that encourages majority rule in government and help strengthen. It's not a surprise it's the case that an open office layout that encourages casual conversations is one of the main tenets of hygge in the workplace.

2. Integrate employee wellness into your benefits package

Every now and then bosses limit their benefits to mandatory time-offs and medical strategies that are imposed from the federal government. The financial compensation of employees should compensate for the absence of worthwhile expansion in employee wellbeing.

This lack of concern for the well-being of employees creates a workplace where employees are constantly struggling with a variety of professional and personal issues. For example, student debt and mental health issues can affect the happiness of employees. Additionally, these are problems that companies can tackle by taking specific measures.

Giving workers-driven benefits like an efficient cafeteria, education cost reimbursement, emotional wellbeing assistance, financial wellbeing and arrangements for childcare as well as other benefits could go a long way to creating a sense of hygge in the workplace.

3. Build the sustainable relationship between employees and their surroundings

Remember that when you work, hygge is strongly connected to the way employees react to and interact with their surroundings. When you work towards the goal of maintenance, you'll be able to create a strong connection between employees and their environment and make them be able to experience "hygge" in the workplace.

Removing paper-based procedures and reducing the need for long trips by providing flexibility and remote working options as well as providing decent food choices are one of the most important steps you can make to create an environment of supportability within the work environment.

Hygge in the beginning of his life

Meik Wiking from the Happiness Research Institute in Copenhagen (and the author of The Little Book of Hygge) acknowledges that there are 10 distinct aspects must be taken into consideration when adopting the hygge lifestyle:

Atmosphere - making a quiet vibe.

The concept of proximity - not having your mobile and living in the moment.

Life should be pleasant, enjoyable and full of joy.

The truth is that no one is better than another.

Friendship Spend time with those whom you cherish and who make you smile.

Appreciation: make the time to think about what you're grateful for.

Harmony - Life isn't an uneasy battle.

Truce isn't a need to argue.

Comfortable - lay back, wear soft socks and enjoy your time.

Asylum - your home is important.

If we accept this as a first stage, I am aware that there are a variety of easy, sensible ways we can integrate the concept of hygge into our design. Here's a list of ideas that you might take advantage of the chance to experiment with:

Try switching your gruelling strip lighting with light bulbs such as pixie lights and LED candles.

Design comfortable spaces where adults and kids can sit down and read.

Bring warm surfaces into your decor, such as sheepskin carpets or sheepskin pads, or woven tosses.

Incorporate nature into your arrangements whenever you can.

You can share the most unforgettable memories you've had all in one place by printing them to frame them with photo albums.

Create small spaces to chat and become one. Include interesting things to these spaces to encourage conversations.

Clean your learning environment so that they appear more comfortable.

Get inspiration from Scandi into the scheme and choose neutral colors such as grays and whites.

Case study: Daisy Chain Nursery

The team at Daisy Chain Nursery has been trying to bring the feel of hygge into their nursery.

A quieting impact

The moment the decision was made to modify the nursery's style The group started by changing the furniture and reducing the music to give the room feel more authentic, and then quickly noticed an improvement in the behaviour of the two-year-olds, as well as children with special needs in their education.

The children appeared more calm and the situation in general seemed to be less chaotic in the sense that children were shut in by their toys and exercises offered instead of being overwhelmed by their surroundings.

The group also noticed that the children were getting settled in faster because a lot of the objects were items they could probably find in their home, and the standard hues were making to make them feel more at ease.

Room in the room

The nursery began the process in the room for infants and started by changing the way work was displayed and purchasing new floor rugs as well as new equipment that would make the room appear more natural.

The plants were familiar with the earth and the normal color materials. Warm white light gathered to create the room a relaxing atmosphere that you could feel as you entered.

The participants used a variety of decorative soft elements and even the teepee with wooden components for exploration.

At that point, they went on to the 2-year-old plan. There was a bit of concern regarding how experts would incorporate the essential integration of the home-from-home method however it was soon established that the process is more about what you can show your children about the things you have , and the impact getting rid of toys could have on children.

The group manufactured a huge sandpit and made it into a natural communication-friendly space, and this has bigly affected the youngsters as they have a safe space to proceed to play where they can utilize their entire bodies.

The addition of more natural resources to the classroom for preschoolers. At first, a significant part of the present decorations was used for the classroom. However the children are right in the process of changing furniture and assets to create a more comfortable space following the purchase of the company's subsequent space...

Ongoing development

In the beginning the group was trying to alter their surroundings by following the home-from-home approach. The nursery they have chosen is an old Victorian home, and the concept of "hygge" fits the design of the building significantly better than a traditional nursery, which is why they had the option of revamping the spaces and make them more welcoming and normal quickly.

Again, this has affected the children, calming their behaviour, and assisting experts to see how they can use the constant education as a tool for learning.

The preschool area in the new location is exceptional when compared with other typical educational settings the group has been made up of to date, showing how the program is continuously improving.

Changes can benefit you.

By utilizing a hygge-inspired approach There are a few basic adjustments we're capable of making to our environment to assist in calming down and enjoying each day. Think about what your children and your group require and, if you decide to decide to try it be sure to take a few minutes to reflect about how the changes are happening and the impact it's having on each of the people who are part of it.

# Chapter 4: Hygge On Holiday

If you look at it carefully the winter holiday season is mostly light-filled holidays that help us through the long, cold winter months to come. However, we then discover ways to ruin the holiday season by worrying about the preparations, the shopping and the food, the guests, the planning and the need for all to go smoothly and have the most enjoyable time ever.

Instead of a holiday splurge there's a holiday war and that's why Hygge comes into play.

Winter is the perfect time to Hygge in Denmark where ever-present winter comes in and people look to soft lighting covers, cosy cups of hot wine to find comfort and pleasure.

In some way or other In the eyes of many, the concept of hygge has evolved into buying the sheepskins of a sack of Oats, but what we're not planning to show you the various items that you can buy. Hygge isn't all about this. It's all about seeing the abundance that already exists to you and organizing it to allow you to enjoy it more. It's about appreciation feelings and simpleness.

Hygge refers to a type of community and care which tends to lose any sense of direction during the fall, as the joys of giving and the shopping madness is a reality. Hygge is snoozing reading a good book in front of the fireplace, enjoying the candle-lit dinner you share with your family, enjoying baking a delicious treat or snuggling on the couch with a loved one or family member beneath a soft cover and just being one.

Here's a list of suggestions you can glance over to help you get the desire. There's no need to try each one of themchoose a few which resonates the most with you.

Give up the world once you step over the threshold. Set up a space where everyone can put their things away or hang up their stuff, even if it means pushing each coat into a pile on the floor in the storage area. Get out of your shoes for the streets and put on the slippers of your choice or thick socks. If you're really serious, dress in your evening robe. The little ceremonies allow you to take a step back from the outside world behind and makes your home seem more like home.

Use roundabout lighting and candles. Give your overhead lighting an opportunity to rest and try making use of more side table lighting. What about all those candles with decorative designs you've put out? Illuminate them at night to take advantage of their radiant glow (securely and obviously). Also, light the chimney if you own one, no matter if it's the end of the week or not.

Set up your furniture in the front room in a way that people can face one another. There's a good chance that your living space is awash with seats and couches that face the television and there's nothing wrong with this. But be aware of the possibility to change a seat to spark discussions. Set a few pads in the ground near the coffee table for someone to crash directly down onto. Try to keep your energy up by standing on the floor more (this is why removing your shoes and wearing slippers can help.)

You should keep at least one tabletop game available. Pre-packaged games are great for cozy, simple and relaxing. Make sure you have at least one entertainment option that is convenient, which entertainment and whatever you find it most suitable for you and your family. Give yourself one less reason to stop playing games with your family.

Let your home smell great. We all have experienced that amazing sensation you feel when you spot something fantastic cooked on the stove, but this is in any way the only method of creating an enjoyable scent. When I was younger my mom used to simmer an aromatic pot on the stove that was heated by wood just for the scent.

Go outside. Walk around. Take part in a snowball game. Once you are in, take a moment to enjoy the feeling of warmness returning onto your face.

Set the temperature of your indoors to lower. Slippers that are fuzzy and comfy socks, you shouldn't perform these hygge-like activities in the event that your indoor temperature regulator is set to levels that are tropical. What's that kind of disavowal regardless? Find out if you're able to take advantage of the advantages of a home that is a little cold and enjoy a lower heating cost while working at it.

Start a tea ritual. Perhaps a wine ritual. Whatever. It's about taking at minimum five minutes to slow down take a drink, relax, and think. For some of us, this is impossible. How do you cut five minutes, the time, place, and how! I'm thinking about it me right now. But, as it happens

I'm in need of it and I'm committing to start this morning.

As a family, we eat together. This is an extreme choice to me as well as my loved ones. Create a plan for December to gather around the table a certain amount of times per week. If you currently do this, congratulations! Continue onward.

Invite people over. Hygge isn't just about engaging in a great way. But, it's closely tied to gathering with the people you love to share a meal or drink. It can be something basic. Maybe it's a slow cooker stew, hot chocolate or popcorn. Don't do it as a favor to start it, just get it started.

Make the occasional cooking ideas simple. If you're one of the people who have to cook dinner late at night , or slamming gaskets to get the powdered sugar onto the desserts perfectly, maybe make it a goal this year to make it less. I've tried this and, my God it's amazing what you can achieve. It's a joy. You'll thank yourself.

Enjoy the beauty of imperfections. When it comes to getting the powdered sugar just right If you're one of those anxious freaks -- and you are because control isn't your thing. one of hairsplitting is denial that the fact that you're a frightbudget Try to let go of it for a while. Find a way to feel comfortable with the unexpected. Snicker at your errors. The flaw is what connects us all to one another. It's when you cease trying to show that you're better than everyone else and admit that you're as flawed. That's the moment you are able to open yourself up to the love and heart that is the spirit of this season. What is more hygge-like than this?

# Chapter 5: What to Hygge

Hygge involves creating an atmosphere which promotes peace and tranquility. It's about accepting things like cakes and having time with loved ones and friends. Hygge is about enjoying the simple pleasures. It is the feeling of comfort or warmth felt when you encounter a particular event, person or setting. That is, the times that makes life worth living. Spending time with friends, family and loved ones is the key to hygge.

The Danes appear to be more modest than other cultures , and Hygge is an integral part of the foundation of Danish society. They enjoy low-cost activities as well as simple pleasures such as drinking coffee and burning candles in order to make a warm environment. Hygge is very popular for Denmark and is a major feature that they use to assess the quality of a Danish party. They talk about events that they are looking forward to and then say that the other wasn't and even mention the great "hyggeligt" (hygge-like) moment was enjoyed by everyone.

Hygge is about the pleasures of living, not things. It could be the glass of wine the fire and wearing comfortable slippers, enjoying dinner with friends, having the chocolate ice cream, or relaxing in the sun with your pet. Spending time with your family and friends is a great way to cozy, and so is taking pleasure in your time off. If you're sitting on the couch with glasses of wine and watch television, you're doing nothing, but you're enjoying hygge. The Danes are cosy like no other country. The typical Danish home is adorned with natural materials such as leather and wood blankets, woolen throws, as well as warm lamps that are strategically placed around the rooms. Lighting is an important element that can bring warmth to the space and help make the room feel comfortable and cozy. Candles are also a common element in Danish homes. They

Danes use more candles per person than any other nation in Europe and higher than the U.S. Alongside feelings of comfort and warmth Hygge is also seen as having benefits for health. It's a sort of Danish variation of the chicken soup. actually a well-known Danish home remedy to treat colds is "tea and Hygge."

By hygge, the Danes have become experts in making the best of things. It was created in response to the harsh winters that last from October through March. In the past, Danes were forced to band with each other to survive the winter and the spirit of community is still in place. The power in our connections is among the main factors that contribute to our mental health and hygge promotes close and more intimate connections.

Hygge does not have any set rules, just general guidelines and suggestions. Everyone has their individual definition of what is comfortable. There are however some rules to help you create the perfect hygge-like atmosphere, in the way that the Danes perceive it. Here are some:

Hygge's flavor is pleasant, familiar and relaxing. You can add a bit of honey to your tea, or a delicious glaze for cookies, or even a hint of wine or your favourite seasonings to stew.

The sound of Hygge is the sound of burning firewood , or sounds like raindrops falling onto the roof, wind outside the window and the rustling of leaves or the creak of the wooden floorboards. Even thunder can be hygge in the case that you're comfy in a warm, comfortable, and relaxing environment when it occurs.

The scent of hygge is one that will take you back to a time where you felt extremely at ease, comfortable and secure. Aromas like lilac vanilla baked goods, wood furniture and a Christmas tree or even your mother's perfume are all examples of hygge.

* The feeling of hygge can be a relaxing feeling that happens when you rub your hands on an incredibly soft blanket, rub your hands with the surface of a ceramic mug or move your hands over the top of an old table.

To experience hygge, you need to take a look at dark, natural hues and observe the slow nature of natural phenomena, for instance, the dance of flames, the fall on snow or raindrops falling across a glass.

The Danish style of living is full of positive aspects and Danes are extremely generous in spirit. Here are some suggestions on how to boost the feeling of hygge within your personal life.

Take pleasure in simple Pleasures

Hygge does not require any of you or require a lot of work. It's about enjoying the precious moments life throws our to our way. When you're reading the comfort of a book with a fireplace, or enjoying a an ice cold drink on the deck make time to be present in the time. Freshly brewed coffee, delicious pastries and sunsets are all part of hygge.

Hygge does not have to mean quiet It can also be about social occasions like eating dinner with a group of people and sharing a table at the local café, or drinking a delicious malty ale in the local bar. Beware, the hygge vibe is infectious. Sooner or later everybody will be doing it.

Reframe Rainy Days

Instead of blaming the cold, winter days take a cue from the Danes and accept the elements. Is it raining? The perfect time to test that new raincoat. Is it snowing? Set the fire. You've been looking forward to starting on a new novel, in all likelihood. Are you not feeling you're ready to go out? Make an easy stew and invite a few guests over for. Hygge is available at any time of the day, at all times of the year. It's a matter of making it happen.

Hygge has a strong association to Danish winters, however it's also important during the summer heat. A refreshing ice cream on a bench in the park or having a glass of beer in the garden is both Hygge. You can count on a candle at the dining table regardless of the weather or season. Candles can be very cozy.

Dress like Danes Dane

Hygge clothing is described as trendy and comfortable. However, it's not unprofessional. In fact, there's no word to describe slobs in Danish since it is not a word that would ever be employed. The best rule of thumb is to wear something bulky but not messy. And should it be cold ensure that you top the look with the appropriate scarf. Here are some important items.

Layers

In any country that has cool temperatures layers are the most important factor to survive the sporadic, ever-changing Danish weather. This is why you should wear a mix of wool sweaters knitted by hand or cardigans and black leggings for girls and dark skinny-fitting black pants for males and black woolen trousers for guys. You're looking for something that strikes an equilibrium between fashion and comfort. Also, always carry an extra layer in case. It's impossible to hygge when it's cold.

Sweaters

It is the ultimate piece of hygge-inspired clothing. The most famous Danish sweater is popularized in the form of Sarah Lund in the Danish TV show The Killing (Forbrydelsen in Danish). Although Forbrydelsen is an Danish show however, The Sarah Lund sweater is not made from it's Danish mainland. Instead, it's an item from the Faroe Islands, which although being part of Denmark is actually towards the north of Scotland and are roughly in the middle of Iceland, Scotland, and Denmark. The sweater eventually was so well-liked within Denmark that the manufacturer could not meet the demand. Faroese sweaters are made using traditional methods and are designed to be worn to serve a practical purpose for protection against winter's cold. Faroese knitwear is manufactured using organic wool that is un-dyed and sourced from the tough northern sheep. Organic wool is more than warm, but it is also light and breathable. It is also hypoallergenic. It is a traditional Faroese sweaters are light in color with dark patterns interspersed into the fabric. They are knitted by hand from an assortment of dark and light wool, and are not dyed with dyes. Their body are made out of the white wool of sheep while the patterns that are darker are created by using the wool of black sheep.

Scarves

In Denmark it is an essential item for females and males. The Danes are so fond of scarves that they're sometimes known as scarf people. The most common rule is large, coarsely woven organic wool, handmade as much as possible, and natural colors. There is also credit if no dyes are employed. The bigger the scarf, the more attractive. Some say that the style is one step away from causing an injury to the neck. Although most people think of a wool scarf as be winter clothes In Denmark the scarf season is from mid-August until mid-June. This means that you will not need a sweater in July. But you can take one just to be prepared in the event that weather changes.

The Color Black

In Denmark the black color is considered to be a primary color in Denmark. After you've left Copenhagen it's possible to feel like you've entered the set of a movie about ninjas. However, while black is the preferred colour for the spring, winter, or autumn, you're permitted to wear more shades in summer or perhaps the gray shade or even wool, when you're looking for something a bit more adventurous.

Wool Socks

Wool socks, just like sweaters and scarves are a must. The Danes regard them as something like hygge-insurance.

Casual Hair

Hygge is all about comfort, simple, and relaxation and the hairstyle of hygge can be described as fashionablely casual, even to the level to be lazy. Make yourself up and wash your hair, trim it if you need to, and then go. These are typically simple cut that is low-maintenance, but slightly messy side, but with just the right amount of mess and incredible. Hygge haircolor is defined by soft, buttery shades that bring comfort and cozy emotions.

Eat Hygge Food

The Hygge food can be described as one of the Scandinavian alternative to comfort food. It embodies the same feeling of contentment and coziness like other types of the term hygge. It is a diet of fresh vegetables and fruits as well as a variety of stews, plenty of delicious buttery desserts along with roasted potatoes, as well as plates of smoked meats as well as wild game and fish. Hygge eating consists of big, easy meals prepared with no disturbance and served with a intimate gathering of your closest family or friends. Sounds deliciously fattening doesn't it? Yet, the Danes are among the most healthy and fit population, with at 21st place in the OECD's weight-loss index over those in the United Kingdom and 26 places less that people in United States. Also, there's not a lot of about yo-yo diets in Denmark. Danes are a healthy people. Danes are able to eat well and manage to do it in moderate quantities.

The sense of comfort we feel from the aroma of freshly cooked meals or baked goodies that emanate out of the kitchen is an excellent way to experience hygge in our lives. It is a reminder of home and takes us back to earlier moments when we experienced similar moments. Foods don't have to be extravagant. They can be cooked out of love. Simple foods such as homemade mayonnaise, roasted beef and potatoes, and homemade bread are especially cozy. I've heard that the less ingredients are in the dish, the less you will have to sacrifice the quality. The care and effort that you place into choosing and cooking these types of dishes contributes to their comfort and hygge.

A Hyggelig Home

Hygge is often associated with feeling secure. A Hyggelig home is warm and welcoming. It provides the visitor with a positive ambience and a sense of belonging. Due to the harsh weather Danes are forced to spend lots of time inside, which is why they invest lots of effort to create a cozy home. The hygge you create in your home is an expression of the energy and emotion you invest in it.

There is an ease in hygge, which lets us enjoy time with family and friends without the need to think of plans aside from enjoying an evening of relaxation. This level of comfort allows individuals the ability to ask questions like "what does it mean to be truly happy?"

You could spend lots of money to fill your home with furniture and other items in a hygge fashion however, without any real feelings behind your choices, your home is bound to have a lack of the spirit of hygge.

Create a Fire

Our ancestors relied on cooking with fire to cook their meals and to keep them and their families warm and safe. In the evenings, they would gather by the flame to cook and eat meals in groups and even slept near the flame. In the end, the fire became an important place of warmth, safety and security. As time passed, this evolved into a society of unity. Nowadays , we hunt in the grocery store and increase the temperature of the central heating system to remain warm. However, those social elements of a social life have been in our human beings' psyche. The idea of gathering with family and friends to share a meal meals is a relaxing event, just like the experience was enjoyed by our forefathers. We can now enjoy the comfort of sitting at our fireplace, while having a good pastry or a glasses of vino. Except if you happen to be going on a camping adventure in which case, by all means create a campfire and take off the marshmallows.

Make Your Own Happy Space

Danish homes are cozy homes that are filled with comfy furniture. Scandinavian furniture is becoming well-known due to its minimalist practical design and focus on natural materials and fabrics. Imagine a comfy leather sofas in a clean living space , adorned with items like sheepskin rugs and plenty of fresh plumped, overstuffed cushions. Research has shown how living in a cozy intimate setting can make us feel happier, as it stimulates dopamine production in our brains, which improves our moods. In effect, Danes have a great hygge fix when they walk through your front entrance.

Be surrounded by Loved Ones

The Danes have a strong culture importance on the concept of community and nothing is more cozy than a cozy gathering with loved ones. When you're living in a country where winters are that are as long and brutal like those you'll encounter in Denmark it can mean the difference between enjoying the moment or being afflicted of cabin fever. Actually, spending time with your family and friends will keep you well-behaved and healthy. So why are you putting off to do? Start a fire, pour an excellent bottle of wine and call your pals an email.

Hygge Music

It is well-known that music affects our mood and can have an impact on our moods and our emotions. The music we listen to is an expression of our experiences and emotions. The lyrics and tunes of our most loved songs usually bring us back to similar events that we have experienced in our lives. we often associate songs with the emotions we experienced when they first came on the scene particularly if it happened in a significant moment of our lives. Studies have shown that music that we feel is pleasing or pleasant triggers the release of dopamine into our brains. This makes us feel happy. However, the reverse could also be the case. Music that is agitated or chaotic could trigger aggressive emotional responses. If we're looking for a relaxing experience, the music we choose to listen to will help to create the right mood.

What does hygge musical sounds like? Much like the word itself, it isn't easy to answer, and the internet can't help much in clearing the confusion. Like the word itself, once you've experienced it, you'll be able to recognize it instantly. A few people appear to view the hygge genre as a word for a ballad or instrumental. As it is, you will see anything including Phil Collins to The Arctic Monkeys or Eminem in playlists with hygge music. I don't claim as an expert on musical styles , but for me personally, these examples do not really convey the essence of the concept of hygge. Hygge, for one, is about creating an atmosphere of shared affection. The majority of songs tend to be a lamentation of the loss of loved ones or regrets. Although these kinds of songs provide a feeling of intimacy, they usually is rooted in hurt -- and is not something we'd want to share with our family and acquaintances. However, there are exceptions to me at the very least the majority of songs about regret or heartbreak aren't authentic hygge-sounds. The majority of hygge-inspired music tends to be peaceful, soothing and peaceful. While there are plenty of loud or energetic songs that bring us happiness, the majority aren't considered to be soothing or tranquil. This means that they don't reflect the true experience of hygge. In the end, the majority of hygge-related music is characterized by coziness, warmth, or comfort similar to the feeling of wearing the woolen blanket or afghan while sitting by the fireplace. But there are songs, no matter how new or old, that give us a feeling of belonging or community, and therefore could be considered to be hygge.

Hygge at work Workplace

We spend at least a portion of our time working like we spend at home, which is why it's as crucial to incorporate hygge into our work environment like it would be to incorporate it into the living space. One way to accomplish this is to fill your home with images of your loved ones and family members or your best moments. Some other hygge-friendly ideas include placing up a photo drawn by child of yours or the kind of cartoon that will make you smile or putting a vase of flowers in a place on your desk. This is a way to inject a little of your home to work so that you can feel relaxed and relaxed while working. Making sure your desk is free of clutter is also an excellent idea since it can help eliminate the sense of chaos that creeps into our lives when we are stressed. Also, warm lighting is as essential in the workplace as it is in your home. Nothing is more unhygge than the bright glow of fluorescent light, particularly in the aftermath of an exhausting day at work.

# Chapter 6: To Relax in Your Home: From Winter Through Summer

Although hygge, in its traditional sense, is about cuddling up to get that warm and feeling good but you can also take it into the summer months. Here's how you can accomplish this:

1. The Flowers

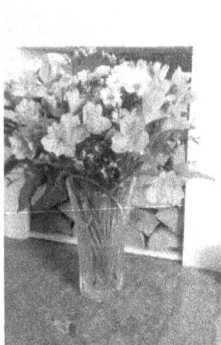

The living room of your home is not going to afford not to have some genuine fresh flowers. According to Danish tradition it is all about simplicity and you don't need to buy the most costly flowers You can also opt for the cost-effective option that is available in your backyard.

Even if you don't want to slash your flower gardens or beds it is the perfect time to use the pruning scraps. Use your imagination and creative thinking tiny branches of flowers can create an impressive look to vase, just like wildflowers that are arranged into beautiful posies could.

If you're having guests over, take advantage of the daisies that are blooming on your fence or lawn with some daisy chains. You can tie them around your vase or use them as wedding rings for napkins, or even string them on your mirror to show off the delicate summer loveliness.

If flowers aren't your thing, there's an alternativeto an arrangement of herbs in a pot. Nothing is better than mint, parsley and basil for this lively cooking in the summer months. It is possible to freeze mint leftovers into ice cubes and add to drinks at night.

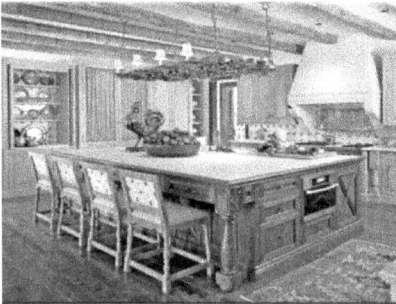

2. Make the Most of the Unique Features of Your Home: Purchase Exposed Beams

The exposed beams that are found in homes are exciting and among the best ways to add character to the simple house. If you're not among the fortunate ones who live in homes that is adorned with exposed beams and you want to know more, make contact with a business like Tradoak as well as other businesses who offer an incredible selection of reclaimed wood beams, which are recycled from beautiful old homes and barns to provide your home with a unique look, no matter how old it may be.

It is possible to improve the look by wrapping some light bulbs around beams, or just hang some terrariums from the ceiling and then plant some small succulents in soil and gravel in order to enhance the new design.

3. Spread The Hygge Feeling to Your Garden

In winter, you have probably neglected your garden. Who would like to sit in the garden to mow in the rain? We're sure you'll agree it is summer the best opportunity to do everything right in your garden. As hygge's all about comfort and warmth, consider your garden as an additional space. It can be very beneficial.

The lighting of your garden can add an element of hygge to your garden, particularly at night. So, think about the cool effect and invest the sun's rays into your garden with solar lights and outdoor lighting. They can be placed in the pathways for the most mystical walk through the garden that every person would want to go on. They can also be placed in areas that you can entertain to keep an inviting glow into the evening.

If you reside in a house you might want to consider windows for your garden. There may not be enough room to entertain however, it's an opportunity to plant plants, flowers, useful herbs, or even better fruit if you're wanting to do something big in a small area outside. There have been great success with strawberries and tomatoes in small pots. You can also plant some cherry plants at the close of summer.

4. Get Cozy

As summer comes to an end it is not necessary to take down your furniture in the garden; purchase weather-proof tables and chairs to give you a reason to enjoy them all year. You can also visit this page to see an online retailer that sells weatherproof furniture. There are ways to make your own comfortable and casual space in your garden that is hygge.

It's as simple as bringing out some pillows and blankets and, in no time you'll be able to transform your garden into a cozy and warm space that can keep the same feeling of hygge in the middle of a cold winter evening.

In the next section, we'll look at ways to integrate Hygge into your workplace.

Hygge All the way to The Office

You can make Hygge moments when you travel to work.

When you are trying to transform to turn your life into a state of hygge one of the toughest aspects is the train or bus (public transportation) journey to work the lengthy, uncomfortable commute. But, you can take action to change this.

If you're looking for happiness, you must be aware that the rules that we live by and the infrastructure of the areas we live in influence and define certain elements of our happiness.

Let's take this for instance: when you work for two hours a day, you have less time at home in your cozy house or eat meals with your loved ones or take part in activities that give warmth and peace. There are some things you can alter but others are not possible to change.

If you can't change something look for a method to handle these issues. One example is when you're taking an train, even though this sounds like a crazy idea it is possible to alter your commute to ensure it is technically longer, to allow you one more stretch to read a good book.

You must create a cozy atmosphere wherever you are. In this instance when you make your commute longer, it indicates that you've created an extra amount of time to yourself. It also means you are able to accomplish something that will make you feel great. Sometimes, the environment dictates the way you commute but you have to figure out your own way to be happy.

In Copenhagen such as Copenhagen which is a city where the majority of people bike into work. You could feel comfortable taking a long bike ride to work If you decide to stay in Copenhagen however it's dependent on your preference for the experience of biking. If you walk to work and that's something you enjoy so much, then you should be Hygge on!

The key is that you must discover a way to make hygge your commute. Let it be simple, but comfortable to let you feel comfortable without worrying about what you're missing in the process. Sometimes the absence of the luxury of a car is a good choice because you don't require it.

For bringing hygge in the workplace, try these things:

1. Own Your Desk

One of the basic Hygge principles is to enjoy the surroundings around you and turning your home into tiny spaces that allow you to unwind whenever you want to.

Therefore, you should customize your office as much as you can, and put an emphasis on the things that enable you to escape the everyday humdrum and spend time enjoying small moments that put happiness to your face and lift your spirits.

Bring photos, your favourite clippings, your favorite mug or other items such as an entertaining comic book to your workplace; this is a great method to bring some personality to your workplace. Many workplace designs are very efficient and rational. To add a touch of hygge to your workplace it is essential to inject some character.

2. Do not leave the outdoors outside

Hygge doesn't just pertain to warm indoor spaces. it is possible to create a feeling of hygge simply by going out to long strolls, looking for wild berries and taking some time to feel the fresh air that hits your skin. It is important to bring a bit of that feeling to your workplace.

In order to bring all those joyous feelings that you feel when you're outdoors, get plants and maintain it when you are at work Plants in the workplace can have a profound effect on the mood at work. Plants can add a bit of energy to the environment with a limited time.

Gather some plants and create an attractive green area within your office. They will be calming and soothing to gaze at.

3: Care for Your Office Lighting

The same light that you'd need on your makeup, is the same light that you require at your table, so that you can write your script. To make the lighting in your office more cozy, it's important to install lamps with warm light (containing an orange tint) throughout the space. Create pools of light- tiny caves of light that you can unwind and enjoy the work.

A table lamp that is suitable to consider is one with a shade that protects the bulb, allowing the light to shine directly on the papers and table without directly shining into the eyes, which is neither ideal for hygge or concentration.

If your workplace allows candles, then you must consider purchasing scented candles. Candlelight, as you are aware, is a source of hygge. However, in general lighting it can bring you closer to the present moment in a unique way. Lighting a candle can be the perfect way to send yourself a message that it's the right time to indulge in Hygge and be immersed in the cozy way.

4: Keep Some Extra Layers

As the winter months begin to set in and the scuffles concerning air conditioning continue to get heated, it's ideal to keep some warm workplace clothes. This could include a vibrant cotton scarf, cashmere sweater, or a pair of socks ideal for those occasions that the rain has washed your shoes to the bone or even a soft cardigan with a cape , which will be the closest thing you'll get to snuggling up in an office blanket.

5: Don't Remain In One Place

Instead of sitting at your desk for the entire day, be inventive with the space around your workplace, and allow yourself to move around to engage in different tasks. In one corner of your room, there are two couches that invite the user to settle down and relax while you work through the script, or while you and your colleague in a conversation.

If you have space to put a couch or a comfortable wingchair you can squeeze yourself into it, consider purchasing at least one of them in lieu of working at your desk for the entire day.

You'll appreciate the cozy feeling that you'll experience when you make your To-Do list, while you are reading your emails or making calls while you drink your cup of coffee on the sofa.

6: Make an Nice Office Playlist

Hygge suggests listening to music as a means to prevent the environment at your workplace from becoming empty or quiet. Get everyone in the office to agree to the radio station, or a great music playlist that includes classical jazz or another type of music that you all be a part of. If that doesn't work, take out your headphones and turn on music you like. Music will always be the key to creating an ideal , hyggelig and cozy environment.

Choose an album of songs that you enjoy and which will create the most intimate and warm feelings whenever you can.

7: Concentrate On Finding Happiness

After you have a better understanding of the meaning behind Hygge, another Danish term that you should add to your dictionary is arbejdsglaede, which refers to "happiness at work.'

In Denmark and in the Scandinavian region in general the job isn't just a means of earning money. Having an excellent level of happiness and satisfaction is something to be anticipated.

Denmark as well as the Scandinavian regions recognize this through flexible work hours, great employee welfare, regular and consistent training (since the Danes like to push themselves to discover new things) or bosses giving less directive orders, so that employees feel more confident.

But, if your workplace doesn't have these things then you could explore your own arbejdsglaede and acclaim others around you by or performing unintentional acts of kindness in your workplace, or having time for yourself every day or having a piece of fruit or two on your desk for you to snack on while working.

8. Make an effort to bond with your coworkers

Hygge can also be defined to be the experience of having the sense of being noticed as a person of significance, and also being in a group of familiar people who make you feel at comfortable. This is the reason why you have to be able to forgive your colleagues.

Start by offering to make your coffee, or ask your coworkers what their day went, or set up regular face-to face feedback session or suggest unique gathering spots - perhaps take one or two of them out to stand up, walk and chat or something similar to that...you are getting the picture isn't it?

It is also possible to organize an enjoyable event for everyone to enjoy as a group. For example, you could visit the downtown café during lunchtime or enjoy some drinks at the local bar after work.

Take note that as you go about this, be sure that you do not appear to be overly intrusive.

As fun shouldn't be confined to the confines of the workplace, you could organize an hour of playtime to play a board game, or any other sweepstake that you want to play you can also suggest time for contemplation during your tea break. The idea of having a intimate chat over a packet of biscuits is an effective way to build bonds with colleagues.

Furthermore, you can set up your food preferences so employees can rotate to bring home-cooked cookies or soups to work. Whatever you decide, remember that it's worth a shot since there's nothing more cozy than creating the time to spend with your friends.

9: Go out for Lunch

In Denmark One of the most snubbed practices includes eating out aldesko. People in Denmark take a break from their work to eat lunch enjoying the outdoors. It's a great option for businesses to set up offices near to the park or walkway. If you are multi-tasking and eating a sandwich while you check your email or type out a message using your computer, you're not living the concept of hygge.

10. Hygge says it's time to go home; show respect This

Don't stay up all night after work. It isn't the way to go. Danes are adamant about their free time and time with family very much. This , combined with their darkness which begins around 4 pm in winter indicates that they are devoted to nothing more than finishing their work in time before heading home to spend the last part of the night with their loved ones.

In the US women generally work about 35 hours a week while men work 41 hours. workers typically work from 8am until 4pm from Monday to Friday. This means they don't enjoy working overtime, or staying late to finish any work left over.

Take on the attitude that is typical of Danes by putting in some long and hard working during the day, and then clocking off at the appropriate time to return back to your comfortable home to rest your body and mind as you dine with your family and friends in a hygge-like way.

# Chapter 7: Art of Decluttering

No matter if you live in a mansion or a small home or even a single room humans tend to accumulate things. It is possible that "things can make us feel happier or make us feel secure or it can be due because objects get more importance as a status symbol, even. In some cases the things we own can distract us from the inner turmoil of us. Feelings of being unfulfilling or feeling of being insecure. Once we have removed the feeling, we are left with ourselves and this is often terrifying.

What exactly does declutter mean? And where should you begin?

Finding Grips by Decluttering

The first thing you should do is take a look around the house. You might be amazed at certain items or objects you're holding onto.

A good example is that painting that was passed down from generation to generation until it eventually, it was hung on your wall, but when you look at it honestly you aren't happy with it. You felt that you were obliged to hang it up because your great uncle, aunt or even your mother gave it for you to be something very unique, and when you got it, you truly felt quite unique.

There's a lot emotions attached to objects. This is why it's vital to think about some guidelines in examining the things you've collected throughout the years, or perhaps just recently.

If you are looking at an object, you should consider:

Does it make you feel happy?

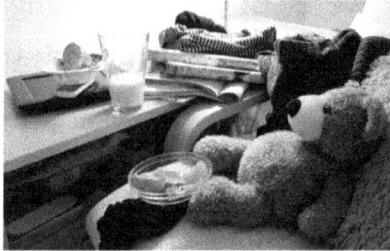

* Does it provide the sensation of comfort and happiness?
* Does it serve some function that is essential to your household?
Is this product able to be placed in a home in which it can reside?
On the negative aspect:
* Does the thing you're looking at trigger intense emotions and feelings inside of you that you would prefer to not feel?
Does the object "in the way is it?
* Does the object have any purpose? If not, then the only purpose was to fill in a gap in the hallway or in a room?

We'll go into more detail about this idea in a minute but this is an excellent place to start. If you are happy with something, hold it. If you're feeling unhappy or unhappy in any way, let the item go. It's not necessary to have the object in your life. Even the memory is long-lasting associated with the object.

A lot of us went to colleges, universities, or went through an era of a frenzied reading and because of this, we accumulated many books. Books are gorgeous and some are more gorgeous than others. The reason you should keep an old book is to go back and read it.

Apart from that the fact that it's to hold onto. Nobody is suggesting you throw your entire library in the garbage. These are just suggestions to assist you in clearing your house and breathing in fresh air and feeling refreshed. The freedom to choose is a key element of hygge.

When ornaments get purchased or gifted as gifts but they aren't helpful, as we certainly don't like them and have no value aside from giving us additional work to tackle when it comes to cleaning the house and as they collect dust.

Another great example to consider when contemplating de-cluttering, is to think about whether the experience or the impression you get from the item is positively or negatively? Photos that are framed to make a statement could trigger a negative emotion in the person. An unhappy divorce could have brought you to the couch you loved, but when you gaze at the sofa, you realize that it is a reminder of the hard times and it's an appropriate time for you to put it down.

If you are unable to decide, storage is a great alternative to get rid of things that we've accumulated that don't serve us or bring us joy. If it is difficult to part with the items, don't push yourself to let go, rather, put the items in a secure manner in the appropriate storage. Every item should be taken care of with care. They were once a source of help for us and might be used by someone else in the same manner. Thus, storing them away is a possibility until you determine what you want to do with them.

Giving things away is extremely Hygge. This is only true when the recipient would gain from the item. The disposal of things should be done with respect. Don't try to transfer things to another person who may be in the same situation similar to you. That is, that oil painting you got from the fox huntcould be as strange to the person who receives it like it is to yourself, however unfortunately , they aren't waking up to the notion that things are meant to please us and, as a consequence, they'll keep it and loathe it the same way you did.

Decluttering should extend to every area in your daily life. Did you ever wear that particular shirt? What about those old pants with two size too large or small?

A lot of people don't like to hear that they're two sizes smaller or bigger! So, get rid of them and be grateful to their time and effort that they were able to serve you. find a pair of trousers that are right for your. The process of dressing will be much simpler and your life will seem easier and you'll be less overwhelmed by the 'tidbits' you manage every day.

The clutter can spread to CDs, DVDs as well as photographs. The piles and piles of photos that are kept in a large black bag will not benefit anyone, not even you.

Explore the photos and select those that are important to you. Display them on your wall or put them in albums that will please you. Remove those that are boring or bring up negative memories. There are a myriad of options today to save photographs on hard drives. The most appealing aspect is that they are incredibly durable. Perhaps this is the approach that you believe is most suitable for you.

Certain people, despite disliking an item or a group of items, may have captured a picture of an object and not kept it to remember the person. There was no reason to keep the watch, lamp made of paraffin, knitted sweater or any other thing. They took a photo of the item instead. It's a simple idea that could aid in decluttering your home.

Some even created wonderfully comfortable cushions out of jerseys they didn't wish to wear, but liked the feeling more than the actual jersey.

Hygge is not a prescriptive concept. There are no do's or don'ts, no rules, or strict guidelines. In fact, they are just suggestions. If you're determined to move into the state of mindfulness that is a peaceful place There are paths to explore to achieve it. It's all about enhancing the Self and improving well-being.

Each step should be completed in a time, and with a lot of thought. Consider how each item within your home can serve your needs or makes you feel good. It's like everything great, it's that it is a process and journey. After the clutter has been cleared and we are left again with our'self' and the things we cherish and love.

# Chapter 8: Be Happy while entertaining

Another way to define the concept of hygge is to avoid those things that make you feel stressed. Anything that drains your emotional energy must be kept away from. Take it off your head. Enjoy the pleasure of relaxing and gentle things. Candles are lit, not just at night, but throughout the day.

As previously mentioned, Denmark has been voted the most happiest nation around the world over the last 40 years. This could be due to the fact that they have the ability to be relaxed and enjoy every minute in their life. Perhaps it is due to the fact that they understand that the possessions of material goods are not required to bring them happiness.

Be less critical of yourself . Learning to be kind to yourself. It will bring you more joy in life . You will also be healthier mentally. Making time for family and friends will give you happier. The most important factor in improve our health is our relationship with one another. Hygge can create more intimate and intimate spaces that are centered around loved ones. A culture that is centered on hygge can lead to families and happy people, and makes a social and community which is extremely caring.

Sipping mulled wine, wearing comfortable pajamas, cuddling cats, and relaxing by a warm fire on a cold evening in the midst of candles; this is hygge.

Baking pastries straight from the oven. Cuddling up to a movie in a blanket of fluffy. Tea is served from your grandmother's old tea table. Family meals with your most loved food items.

Hygge means coziness in translation, but it's actually far more.

Denmark is a country with very long and cold winters. It is a country with bad weather for the majority of the year , and has the 17-hour period of night each day in winter , and temperatures that hover around 32°F. The majority of people are inside. This is the ideal opportunity to entertain.

Hygge might be dining with your family or friends. It could be spending peace and quiet reading your favorite book, unaffected. The mood is set by creating small, cozy areas for guests to snuggle together and enjoy themselves. Hygge's main idea is to feel at home and relaxed. Let go of all the worries of the world.

The Danes have known the secrets of hygge since the beginning of time. Relaxing and having a cozy time with family and friends over a cup of coffee, cake and a beer, is extremely relaxing for the soul. Hygge is a way of being nice to yourself. Do indulge, but don't let yourself down, have an enjoyable time and don't be a slave to yourself. This is helpful when people are trying to eat healthier and exercise throughout January while abstaining from drinking alcohol in the course of all the New Year's resolutions.

Danes don't deny their own existence. Danes are kind to one another. There is no talk of eating disorders or eating problems in Denmark. They don't understand the meaning of the yo-yo diets. This is the primary reason for their happiness. the U.S.

If your guests leave after having a great moment, you could receive an acknowledgment of having had an enjoyable and hyggelig time.

Hygge isn't just for those who are wealthy. Everyone can enjoy it, from the wealthiest to the smallest. Hygge is a must for the Danish.

One of the closest English word to hygge in the English language that is similar to hygge is hug. The benefits of both are quite like. They are both extremely comfortable and secure. As per the Oxford English Dictionary, the definition of hug is "to be a lover of oneself or to make oneself comfortable".

There are many cultures that have expressions that are like the concept of hygge. Germany has Gemutlichkeit, which is a feeling of health and well-being that is based on great foods, friendly company and a drinks. Danes believe that hygge's characteristics are completely exclusive to them.

The word "hygge" isn't meant to be transliterated. It needs to be felt. The concept is rooted in the concept of social democratic system. Nearly everyone who isn't Danish descent has trouble understanding the significance of social relations.

Get your drink of choice or glasses of vino. Set off an fire. It doesn't matter whether it's outdoors or inside. Invite your guests over, spread out the blankets and relax with your friends. Chat about your week, day, or even the entire year. Keep in touch. And most importantly, be happy with the company of others.

Here are some ideas to help you get going. Have a pie for dinner. Have a glass of wine. It's totally guilt-free. If you are hosting a party, you're able to wear your scarfs. Get your shoes and wear them. Warm your favorite pair jeans in the dryer , then put them on as warming. Bake your cake and invite a guest to join you for a meal. Why? Simply because. Pour a cup of coffee on. Use two forks to eat the cake, then the coffee, to the flame with the candles lit and then eat the entire cake while laughing, talking and having a good time in the Hygge.

Candles are a crucial part of the hygge effect. Danes can burn approximately six kilograms of candles per year. This means that each person has to burn around six kilograms of candles. This is not the whole nation, just each and every one. Danes even carry candles when they go on vacation.

Hygge for me is a peaceful family get-together. There would not be any discussions about the problems the family members were facing political, or about who was on the honor roll or what the family is currently working. No rudeness, no negativity, no complaining. Everyone is there to help. There is no one who gets to do every task. Nobody competes to see who is more successful. No one attacks anyone other than themselves. No bragging. It's a simple interaction with the emphasis on food, people, and the enjoyable moments. It's a place to hide from the world outside.

Some people think this could be a typical gathering. But for the majority of us, it's not.

Here are some easy rules for an event that is hygge:

Be yourself. You don't have to wear a snazzy outfit. Simply be yourself. Keep your guard up. You're not likely to be assaulted at a gathering of hygge and no one will try to harm you. The use of boasting, resentment and competition are all ways to divide, not uniting.

Do not get caught up in the controversy. If you select an issue that is controversial there isn't an atmosphere of hygge. Hygge is a calm debate flow. Be in the present. There is a place for argument within the everyday routine. Hygge is about enjoying your food and the company of others. Negative, complaining, judging and arguing are not permitted in a cozy environment.

Join the team. Everyone will be able to think of ways to assist, without needing to be requested. This helps keep the flow smoothly and everyone has all the work to do. When everyone contributes to the drinking, serving and cooking, Hygge will blossom.

Hygge is a refuge from the world outside. Hygge is a refuge from the pressures of competition, materialism social networking and climbing. It is the time when everybody can relax and share their thoughts without worrying about being scrutinized. It's the time and space in which all things are sacred, and any issues are put aside. This allows family members and friends to get to know each other without having to worry about being assessed.

The time for this is short. Hygge can be a challenge for anyone who isn't Danish. There is no negativity and no one is bragging or complaining, nobody is trying to dominate the on the stage, and nobody is in a debate. This is not possible for the majority of families. The reward is amazing. It's great to share these moments with the people you cherish. If you realize that you are only sharing it for a brief period this makes it simpler to be able to cherish every minute.

The memories you have left behind will remain with you even after you go. For the present time, they'll be fine outside , so you can spend a fantastic time with those you cherish.

# Chapter 9: The Way That The Hygge Lifestyle Could Help You Save Money

It's a good thing that hygge actions like clubbing or eating out, or shopping will also be different in purposes of all kinds They're expensive. Hygge-related activities, however generally, are minimal or even cost-free. The lifestyle of hygge as the ideal choice for those who want to live an enjoyable lifestyle while adhering to an extremely tight budget.

As with any other designs, hygge may be blamed for helping sell costly products. Charlotte Higgins, composing for The Guardian, discusses seeing Hygge "used to sell cashmere sweaters background, wine for a veggie lover's shepherd's pie, sewing patterns and a skincare product and small bridles with bubbly for dachshunds, yoga withdrawals as well as an event in a "shepherd's house" located in Kent." There's also plenty of books you can spend your money on to become familiar with the lifestyle of hygge.

In addition to that be, in the end it's not about things. As every story emphasizes the fact that it's about an mental state or inclination that you cannot acquire simply by spending money. The truth is, "futurist" Lucie Greene addressed to the New York Times, ventures to the point of to describe the hygge style as in response to the prior "prosperity growth" that seemed to focus upon "$100 Lululemon tights and $10 Jugs of cold squeezed juices."

The way of living that is hygge However, it is also within everyone's reach. As with the deliberate ease of development is centered around stepping off, taking on nature, and creating more opportunities for friends Everything you can handle without spending any cash at all.

Hygge Lifestyle Benefits

Do you like squeezing in with a bookcase, some coffee and some good books? There is a chance that you could be practicing

Hygge more often than you think. Hygge is a concept that was born in Danish culture that focuses the importance of living with a sense of peace, comfort and peace. Hygge has been described as "making an environment that is warm and gaining a sense of the positive aspects of life with wonderful people."

There's a debate about the best method to describe the concept of Hygge or, more specifically "tone the guh" as well as "hoo-gah," however what is interesting about these concepts is the fact that there are actual health benefits associated with continuing living a Hygge-focused living.

The benefits of Hygge

There's been a myriad of benefits associated with the practice of Hygge. Scientists have found that satisfaction researchers consistently find Denmark to be one of the most happy people on Earth and this is something that Danes believe is due to the activity of the hygges. The feeling of joy growing is certainly a benefit of practicing Hygge but there could be more physical, energetic and emotional benefits too.

Enthusiastic Benefits

Hygge style is a concept to create a sense of peace and harmony in the living area. Because we are aware of the way we interact and experience life through hearing, sight, touch with taste and smell It shouldn't be a surprise to person that creating a comfortable living space can help people to feel less than an edge and give us feelings of intense well-being and prosperity. This feeling of comfort and security could more easily allow us, and them and also the space that they offer to us, to lay go of our barriers and become ever more open and present to connecting with others.

Possible examples of benefits that could be passionate might include:

There is less worry and sorrow

Increased self-esteem and confidence

Positive thinking that is expanded

Pressure was reduced

The most notable feeling of care

Self-empathy developed

Accompanying act that is expanded

Physical Benefits

At the moment we feel a sense of calm and security the body responds according to the needs. It is when we perceived danger or risk that our bodies usually respond with combat, flight or even freeze. Hygge is a state of mind that creates an environment of relaxation and comfort, where our bodies and psyches become more relaxed. In this kind of space there is less need to be concerned about our state for signs of danger.

Possible physical benefits might include:

Restorative improvement

Weight guideline

The cortisol (stress hormone) increases

Self-care can be improved

Requirements for less risky adaptation practices such as liquor or medication

Hygge Social Benefits

When we feel comfortable and secure, we are bound to build and strengthen groups with others. In the hygge-centric way of living has a focus of interacting with your families, friends, and families. Spending time with those who are important to us created the feeling of belonging to an area and a group that is constantly revealing affects our well-being and happiness. We feel more secure when we're with others We feel the feeling of being secure to venture out on our own and are more open to the possibility of rehearsing our feelings of powerlessness with people around us, and which can be facilitated in the hygge-style home.

Possible social benefits might include:

Focus on the fellowship

The sighs of peace and tranquility

Trust that is expanded

Closer and more intimate

New social organizations

New connections are improved

A lesser dependence on web-based networking media

How to use Hygge in Your Life

Many of us want to feel at peace, calm and comfortable however do we have to relocate to Denmark in order to fully understand the Hygge way of living? Not really! There are a myriad of ways to integrate elements of hygge in our daily life and living spaces. Implementing some of these aspects can begin giving you that feeling of harmony, community and comfort throughout your day-to-day life.

Lighting

Lighting is an essential element that creates a feeling of hygge within the living room. The use of soft, warm white light creates an appealing and cosy space when contrasted by stark, stunning fluorescent bulbs or white bulbs. Remember that the more lumens of the bulb, the better the lighting. You can also add a dimmer to provide options for lighting your space in how you wanted to.

Other options are to utilize floor lamps instead of overhead lighting. Above lights can produce lighting that is insanely bright for the space and can appear like a place of authority. With the use of table and floor lights, consider lighting to make a space that is more private and lighting zones in which people are seated to read or unwind, and talk to each other.

The truth is that candles are a signature light employed in a hygge style space. Candles create an ambiance of warm, soft light and provide a sense of solace and relaxation that are widely admired in this type of style. If candles that are open flamed pose the greatest danger to your home due to pets or young children, you may select candles with LEDs.

Surface

Hygge is all about things that feel soft and cozy. It is important to combine delicate ornamentation like hurls, spreads cushions, and floor coverings to create a cozy and inviting area. The soft surfaces help to relax and help us be relaxed when stress levels are intense. The sensitive surfaces allow others to feel that everything is well within the space in calming anxiety and encouraging people to have fun to one another. Exchanges can feel calm and relaxed in this environment instead of feeling overwhelmed or restricted.

Formal format that is expressive

A peaceful environment can be created with the use of ornaments such as wooden parts or indoor plants. They can also be used in a fundamental simple, minimalist style. Try to select items that are of a high-value such as photographs of your loved ones or family. It is possible to place photo collections on the table, with images of growth or memories which you've shared with other people. Hygge is all about intimacy and warmth So use a bold design to entice people and create conversation.

Warmth

Warmth isn't a huge quantity of temperature, as it's an indication of a spirited warmth. A stack is the most recognizable characteristic of a space that is hygge-inspired however it's not a possibility for everybody. Whatever you do to create an comfortable, warm and inviting space will at least be an. The most common examples of this are candles and also shows how to use them to complements lighting. It is also possible to make use of small string lights to illuminate specific areas of your home to create that captivating warmness that fireplaces could bring to the space.

Shading

The colors that are picked by professionals are an essential part of creating a welcoming space for you and your guests. The most popular colors are neutral particularly the delicate whites reddens and delicate Tans. The usage of neutral colors on the wall can really assist to calm your mind that is in keeping the particular style of living. Hygge is all about calm moderate, sensitive and calming. In a way Hygge is the fad of uncomfortable living conditions and spending time with your close friends, loved ones and family.

The Individuals

Connecting with other people is the very heart of living in a hygge style. The goal is to be open and connected with those in your vicinity. Through maintaining these connections, you are enabling yourself and others to feel a sense of belonging. When we feel are aware that we have a home that we are in, we experience a sense of passion and wellbeing. A sense of security that is passionate can create a positive social experience and lets us experience the physical benefit of simpleness as well as quietness and connection.

Action

Hygge-style activities typically contain things that aid in feeling calm, comfortable and connected to other people. Social gatherings with friends at home are a must. The social events revolve around the connection with other people rather than the introduction. There isn't any requirement for a proper black tie affair. In truth, hygge living suggests the opposite. Gatherings should be a place that is comfortable, welcoming and provides people with a place to be in awe, and concentrate on the bonds and relationships with each other. Think about a game night with colleagues, inviting friends or friends over for coffee, or to encourage to have a book club.

The most efficient method to utilize Hygge at Work

It is possible to without much of an effort create hygge-inspired areas in your work space. It is in the workplace that you may find yourself feeling difficult to manage ourselves, or keep a situation one that is centered on peace and harmony. Find a few, easy methods to manage adjustments to your environment to promote a feeling of peace. You'll believe it's simpler to recognize the value of your space, which can bring more benefits and increase satisfaction for your business.

Ideas to try:

Highlight light that is delicately white light

Little-trimmed succulent plants

A floor covering for the measured area to cover your workspace

Pictures of family members

Hygge is about relaxation and harmony as well as connection. The advantages of doing some of these aspects are a result of our passion for well-being, physical health and our social well-being. Integrating some of these concepts to your daily life could give you a place that is a relaxed, warm and welcoming to others and extraordinary for your health and well-being.

Ten Top Tips to Manage the stress

For some, the joy and happiness of the holiday season can lead to an uneasy and busy January. With tensions from the New Year's resolutions and working after winter festivities, many workers are feeling stressed and anxious during January.

The International Stress Management Association offers the following suggestions for managing stress so you can start the new year with a sense of confidence and in control:

1. Make yourself the first priority by eating nutritious meals as well as scheduling physical activities that you like, and managing your time effectively. Prioritizing your needs puts you in a position to assist others.

2. Begin organizing tasks. Select your three most important tasks each day and turn them into a necessity. Reschedule, negotiate or delegate tasks which don't meet the criteria.

3. Start to take time to relax and relax. Think about ruminating for a few minutes each day to ease anxiety and strengthen your secure structure.

4. Begin to establish a connection with other. Be aware of your fellows' communication styles and strive to solve problems by working together.

5. Start making every second count. Be aware of what you've got. When you do this you can new opportunities for development and learning.

6. Quit overlooking your needs. Pause for a few minutes throughout the day. Know when and when to say 'no' both at work and at home.

7. Eliminate unnecessary interruptions. You might want to ask your partner as well as your family members to assist in organizing what tasks are important and which chores should be put off.

8. Stop allowing people to feel inferior. Accept yourself for who you are. Take advantage of past mistakes and concentrate on your strengths which are good for you.

9. Quit being critical. A flexible reasoning style that combines being targeted and

understanding will increase your mental health.

10. Take a break from keeping a distance from the things you don't have to complete. When you delay them you put them at the forefront of your mind , and they become more important. Make sure you are in control and give yourself a prize once you've completed.

How to Obtain Danish Happiness

Hygge is in essence a non-dramatization harmony time. It's relaxing in or "at the hygge signature," in any case and more it's a constant reminder to the fact that it is sacred and observing it in this way.

Because Danes believe that hygge is in that role as an integral part of living a happy life and they work in tandem to make it happen. Hygge can be described as "we the time" rather than "personal time" Hygge is viewed as an incredible element of Danish joy that some institutions across the UK and in the US are now offering classes on the subject.

Many people think about lighting candles, preparing delicious food, and creating the most of a pleasant climate. However it's just the surface of the concept of hygge. In actuality it's that it is much more than that.

What is hygge exactly? Try to imagine going to a non-dramatization family gathering. There is no tense discussions about legislation and family problems or Aunt Jenny's naughty children.

There is no grumbling, angry remarks or a soaring resentment. Everyone helps to ensure that nobody is unable to complete the task at hand. There is no boasting, attacking anyone or fights with anyone else. It's a jolly balanced, tolerant group which is focused on creating a positive impression aside from all other things including the food and the business. In simple terms an oasis away from the world.

For some, this might sound like a typical gatherings with family members.

However, for the majority of us, however, it's not. The implicit principles of hygge are what makes it an exceptional experience. American Anthropologists who have looked at Danish hygge are stunned by the simple flow in the hyggelig world of communication, and the way that nobody tries to become the primary center of attention. This is a brief moment in which everyone takes off their veils and sheds their worries and ask to be a part of the high quality of life and connect with other people. There is a wealth of research to show how important social connections are to success.

The feeling of being a part of something can give meaning and significance to all aspects of our lives. Social connections can increase the length of life, reduce stress and can even improve our fragile framework. By committing time and energy to "hygge" we can create an environment that is safe for family members and friends to live together and with no stress. In the end it is a matter of everyone needing for this to work together in order to achieve it.

Scientists also discover that Denmark's libertarianism plays an important role. For instance, a new study by Robert Biswas-Diener and co-workers found that although wealthy Americans as well as Danes were equally happy however, the true result was that low-paying Danes were far happier than their American counterparts. This is backed up by research that has shown that show significant levels of balance change into more joyful social order. Naturally, libertarianism is an integral belief of Hygge, according to the anthropologists. Perhaps, in this way the norms that govern the private life of Denmark transform into the kind of open additions referred to by Bernie Sanders.

Here are five tips to hygge that you may have to incorporate into your lifestyle.

1. You are who you appear to appear to. Be yourself. Your genuine self. Don't let your watchman go. You won't be slapped on the Hygge turf, and you won't be a victim. When we are no longer trying to prove something, we'll be able to all identify with a more authentic way. Glamour, rivalry, and misrepresentation aren't holding and separating, but rather, unpretentiously securing.

2. Do not be deceived by the debate. If your idea is overly authentic and controversial the chances are it's not an ideal hygge. Hygge is about a and synchronized exchange of information in a positive manner. The focus is on being moment and staying on the right time. There is a lot of moments in our everyday lives to engage in debate and argument. the experience shows that hygge can be closely tied to getting an energy boost from food and organization and not being involved in matters that hinder that. So, complaining, arguing as well as judging

and arguing aren't permitted in the hygge environment.

3. Consider yourself a coworker. Everyone is aware of what the individual who is in question has to contribute without asking questions. This makes the whole flow more efficient and no one gets trapped doing everything. When everyone is able to cooperate in preparing for serving, pouring, and as well as chatting and chatting, Hygge has exploded. In any case, everyone should realize that they're a small part of the group.

4. Hygge is a place of refuge all things taken into consideration. Hygge time is associated by offering a temporary shield from social climbing, system administration, rivalry and real-world realism. It is a place where everyone can let loose and be open to their souls without judgement regardless of what's going on in their lives. For good or awful, this space is a holy place where concerns can be left out.

They are unique in the sense that they take into account family members and friends to always have the possibility of collaborating in this area without fear of judgement.

5. It is a time-bound. Hygge is a good idea to try to be a more non-Dane. No one is constantly the focal point, nobody complaining or complaining, nobody having a negative attitude and everyone trying to stay calm and avoid any belligerence? It is a challenge for many families! However, the end outcome is awe-inspiring. It's a daunting thought to spend these free minutes with the people you care about. In the event that you know that it's only for a meal or lunch or limited time frame this helps to really try to enjoy the minute.

Your troubles will be hanging close to you from the entryway to hygge's after you have left. However, for the duration of a few minutes, they'll be able to wait outside for more important things.

# Chapter 10: The Hygge State of Mind: How to Have The Hygge Mindset

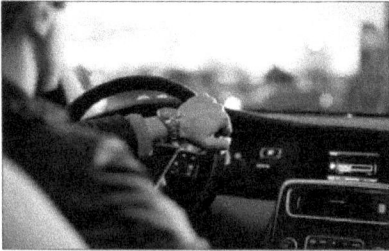

Hygge is becoming more and more fashionable across The West as a trend in lifestyle. It's not just an item on a shopping list or style of decoration. It's a way to live living. It's a way of thinking.

Hygge is all about enjoying an intimate candle-lit meal with your family and friends. It's about snuggling with your beloved with a warm blanket. It's about sitting outside on your patio while watching the sun set. It's more than an overwhelming sensory experience. Hygge is more than just the comfort and cosiness. Hygge is an art of appreciation for the beauty in all of the small things. It's about having gratitude in your heart. Here are some helpful tips you can follow to attain "hygge the state of your mind".

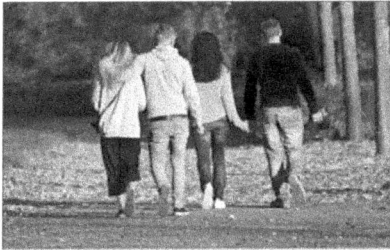

Choose to focus on the positive
Denmark is a gorgeous country. It's awash with pastel-colored buildings. It is a paradise for beach lovers as well as fascinating cityscapes and stunning landscapes. It's stunning in summer months. However, it is too cold in wintertime. However the Danish people make the most out of winter by engaging in hygge.

Hygge isn't only about being comfortable or cozy. It's about having positive attitudes. It's about focusing on the positive side of every circumstance. This is about having a half glass full type of guy.

Slow Down

We live in a bustling world. We are multi-tasking, we consume quickly, and strive to achieve our goals. This is why a lot of us are stressed and depressed.

It is about slowing things down, and living in the present. It's about making unforgettable memories with loved ones. It's about taking your time.

Here's how to speed up your pace:

## 1. Do less.

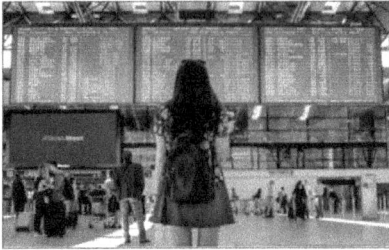

Don't be ashamed to do less. Eliminate actions that aren't in line with your objectives. Don't get lost in meaningless busyness. Choose activities that make you smile and bring you joy and make your heart jump.

2. Take a break when you need to.

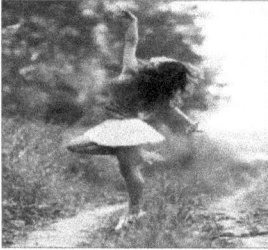

Work and play can make your life seem unstable. Therefore, do yourself a favor by taking time off. Relieve yourself when you're tired.

Relaxation boosts the immune system. It helps you feel more energetic and improves your overall health. It can also slow down the process of aging, and boosts your productivity and creative.

3. Do a digital detox every now and every now and.

Electronic devices allow us to communicate with loved ones even when they're not around. However, they are often distracting and could reduce your efficiency. Make sure to turn off your phone when working on something important, so you can concentrate.

Enjoy a weekend getaway with your special someone. Put your phone down and enjoy the time with your loved ones. Don't answer calls. Don't share any content on Instagram. Don't check your Facebook.

4. Get in touch with nature.

Nature has a way of being simply appealing. It energizes your soul. Instead of heading to the gym, take a hike instead, and stop to be awed by the wonder and beauty of nature.

5. Do not try to multi-task.

Many people believe that multi-tasking is a key to boosting productivity. True to some degree. But, it is possible to make you feel tired and hinder your focus and mental focus. To lead a tranquil life, focus on only one thing at a.

6. You should drive slower.

It is safer to drive slowly and also provides you with an time to relax and enjoy the ride. It's the perfect opportunity to take in the sights from your town.

Also, make sure you take a mentally healthy day off, at minimum once per month. If you're feeling exhausted, stressed or feel that you're on the verge of breaking down you can take a few days to yourself. Go to the movies or read a book or go to the nearest beach.

# Chapter 11: Tips to Enhance Your Home and Lifestyle

Relaxation and Comfort

Hygge is about feeling comfortable It is a time to relax away from everyday routine. It's a time to unwind from the daily stress, pressures and busy schedules. One of the most essential aspects of Hygge is creating a space and a space that is relaxing for you.

To create an Hyggelig environment, we must focus more on harmony and balance rather than just display so rather instead of accumulating too many items to create a comfortable atmosphere it is important to select items that mean something to us and that we are passionate about the things we love. One of the ways to care for things is giving the space to breathe, and keep the space free of clutter. It is important to place in our surroundings only those things that tell our personal story, our beliefs and things that we are connected to. In such a setting you'll discover peace, inspiration, and tranquility.

Atmosphere

It's an attempt to create a Hygge ambience. You should be in a space and dressed in a way that encourages coziness and comfort.

The Hygge spot

What part of your home (it could be your home in a hotel room, office, or home) are you most comfortable ? It could be a window in which you can cover yourself with a cozy blanket, kick your feet on the floor (maybe) and let the world pass through your window. It could also be your rocker of choice by the fireplace that you can curl in a cozy book. It could be a couch on which you are able to cuddle with your loved ones, wrap yourself in a cozy blanket, enjoy popcorn while watching the latest television series. If it gives you that sense of comfort, it's a good idea whatever it is. In Danish the term for your cozy spot is known as the Hyggekrog.

Hygge Clothing

You need to wear comfortable clothing. It can be anything, there is no need to be dressed up for this event. It's funny, the majority of our comfortable clothes, the ones we cuddle on the sofa with during the weekend or on evenings are the ones we'd never wear in public. These are the clothes that we're talking about. Actually, there's an Danish term that describes it as Hyggebusker.

Lighting

It is possible to turn off your overhead light and put out candles. If you inquire with the Danes to explain that without candles, there's no Hygge. It is possible to enter an Danish house and think they're not wealthy enough to have the "standard lighting" that we're used to however this isn't the reality. They favor candles because they see them as the most essential element in creating a Hyggelig environment.

Twinkly Lights

They're bright and festive and would look wonderful anywhere, in your patio, bedroom, or even in your bathroom. They are perfect for Hygge lighting because they emit a soft lighting, much like candles. They also look attractive but without becoming excessive.

Warmth

A blanket that is warm It is essential to have a blanket to wrap yourself around. It should be cozy and comfortable. It could be a padded blanket or a chunky knit or even a heated throw blanket, but it needs to be one that you enjoy (we each have a favourite blanket that gives an ideal hug along with warmth).

The fireplace there is a fireplace in your house make use of it to create a Hyggelig environment. Imagine yourself reclining in front of the fireplace in the cold winter evening, sipping something sweet and warm. It's extremely cozy isn't it. It's part of the Danish tradition of gathering around the fire. It can be within the home (fireplace) or set it up outside (as for bonfires).

Home Decor

The decor of a home that is hyggelig should reflect the warmth and comfort. For example, decorating with soft comforters and fluffy pillows with warm colors like mustard and bright green can make your home feel more comfortable and comfortable.

Color is an integral part of interior design. The colour scheme of your home is crucial also when it comes to Hygge. It shouldn't be excessive. It is important to keep the space cool, warm and most importantly , simple. A neutral color scheme will be ideal for creating a room a sense of calm and peace. To create an Hygge color scheme, think about the following pastel hues: lighter greys, browns, and cream.

Additionally, there is the texture. It is not something we think about when creating the Hygge environment. But, it's important to be aware of this when we design our home decor. Imagine having warm and soft texture within your living space. Consider natural warm materials like hardwood flooring for your floors as well as kitchen countertops and tables. Additionally, you can use wool for throw blankets flooring rugs, clothing and blankets. Isn't it warm and cozy as you walk around or gaze at? The combination of texture and color creates the appearance of warmth and comfort.

Bathrooms Hygge spa-like bathroom

The bathroom is a space to cleanse your body using water and soap, but also to be an area of peace where you can breathe deep breaths, take a break and reenergize. It must be cozy, warm and relaxing.

Don't forget the short showers early in the day. Get your shower earlier so you have time to unwind. The ambience in the shower is also important. Set off some candles that have your preferred scents and alter the lighting. Remove the unnecessary items that might otherwise clutter your bathroom. For added pleasure, get yourself some warm robes that you can cover up the warm bath.

Indulgence/Pleasure

It's a perfect the midst of a moment to take a breath and enjoy the joys of life. you are now ready to indulge in an indulgence. Treat yourself to a tasty meal We're talking about cakes, sweets or savory dishes. You can also enjoy hot drinks. You can even have sweet wine, if you're into it.

In Hygge is the right to indulge in some of your favorite foodsthat many of us aren't allowed to eat. You are trying to create a warm feeling, and the food you consume has an important part to play in it. You know, the kinds of food that makes you feel cozy and happy do you not?

While you indulge your self without limit take note that Hygge is a mode of restraint which means that there is no excess eating or alcohol consumption because there isn't any Hygge in drinking or binge eating It's all about moderateness.

Application

There's no need to shell out money for these meals. If you can prepare them at home, then the more convenient, since the goal is to increase your comfort and comfortability. For Danes this could include making cakes coffee, hot chocolate, or even pastries. In other regions in the world, many stick to their traditions; some even copy the Danes while others create whatever they feel like even if it's chicken soup. There is no limit with regards to the food choices for comfort.

The Sense of Togetherness

Humans have a social nature, creatures It's part of our DNA to be a part of a community. If we're alone or do not have loved ones around us, we're not achieving our totality. Healthy relationships are vital to our happiness as well as our health.

In a state of overwhelm by our hectic schedules, it's easy to lose track of relationships and forget the importance of one another. Individualism is a popular concept within our culture. Personal interactions are now limited by social media and chats. video and text messaging that are available across the globe have been gaining popularity. The people have learned to set aside their personal relationships, to be in solitude and pursue the material riches. But the truth is that nothing can ever be able to replace the warmness of social connections. We're trying to change the things that are already part of our DNA. Human beings are social creatures, period. The latest ideas about what we ought to be doing in our lives are not going to change this fact.

This does not mean that we have to sacrifice our personal identity and surrender in our friendships. In Hygge the individual is also important however there is a sense that without the involvement and support of others , which can lead positive relationships we will never be truly content as a person in its entirety. as a whole (the human being who socializes) is dependent on the support of others.

Whoever first conceived of Hygge realized that relationships play a major role in our wellbeing. The concept of being together is an integral part that is a part of Hygge and vice the reverse. It is evident that through Hygge we are able to establish and develop strong bonds with others. What is Hygge's purpose? might be wondering. Let me explain:

The best relationships are formed by spending time together. If all you do is be nice to one another for a short time while you try to keep up with your hectic schedule relationships will be strained and never be able to grow. It is essential to spend time getting to get to know your partner and share stories food and laughs as well as to have fun together and share the joy of friendship.

Hygge allows spending time with family and friends engaging in all of these activities to be easy, smooth and free of everything that could affect your mood negatively, such as expectations. It is easy to be in Hygge because in its simple and relaxing setting it is possible to spend time together with loved ones and not have any elaborate plans (such as expensive brunches, or dinners that are generally thought to be more enjoyable) apart from just sitting back and enjoying your time with them.

In this context we are able to be who we really are and be ourselves, something that's difficult to do when you're with everyone. The best company can give us an assurance of security than having people who accept usfor who we are, and with people who are not required to conceal the person you are. This means that we are in steady relationships and can never be lonely, regardless of the circumstances. It's a wonderful source of joy.

Being together can make Hygge more enjoyable and enriches the experience. Hygge experience more enjoyable and wealthy! It's about having fun with the little things in life and helping each other to discover the strengths and weaknesses of each other and working together to bring out the best. It is essentially the teamwork of all people and no one needs to be feeling alone.

Application

Take time to spend time with those who you cherish or with whom you have in common. It is possible to do these things: travel with your family and friends, enjoy good food with good company, relax at home with your family and friends Take dancing and cooking lessons, or work on a project that inspires you with people who are similar to you and so on.

Equality and Harmony

The concept of "togetherness" wouldn't be a good fit for Hygge in the absence of equality and it was not in harmony. If you're spending time having fun Hygge with your friends it is important to have equality everywhere. It's time to share chores, time, and space. If food needs to cook, you can help each other out in the kitchen. In the event of storytelling, all is involved in the storytelling, and if there's the possibility of watching a program all should be in agreement with the show.

Hygge is all about creating a sense of equality in which there is no distinction between people or arguing in Hygge time. At this point it is vital to create a space where everyone can be equally valued. That means that there should be no boasting about achievements and discussing topics that matter to everyone. It is also helpful to spend time with people who already enjoy us. People whom you don't have to impress. Be aware that you should feel relaxed, relaxed and not putting on a show.

The Presence

Are you constantly contemplating past events? Do you worry about the future, arguing and fretting about the things you're working toward? If you're often unhappy most likely, you've allowed these thoughts such as your past and future take over your life. One thing you've missed is that you are in the present moment in the present moment.

The ability to be present is an important aspect of Hygge. It is impossible to relax and enjoy the warmth of the midst of a Hyggelic evening if you are caught up in your thoughts is stuck in the past or the future, and unable to be present in what's happening right now. To truly be in Hygge you must be able to enjoy the present moment and appreciate the warmth and pleasures in the present.

A popular Hygge clichés is to curl up with a blanket in your favourite seat while reading a book and sipping hot chocolate on an icy winter night. Anyone can enjoy this environment, and leave as exhausted as they are or more. What makes Hyggelig distinctive and effective in providing peace, relaxation and tranquility is simply being present in that moment, reading a book and enjoying the flavor of the hot chocolate as well as the warmth of an evening that is cold. It's the enjoyment of the whole experience that can make all the difference.

Application

Being present present is a practice you can develop. If you're doing the same thing of drifting off in your thoughts and being unhappy, this is what you will always be. If you wish to be in Hygge then you must get your mind trained to be fully present. What can you do to achieve this? Let's discover the answer.

* Turn off the phone.

If you are having your Hyggelig experiences, make sure to keep your phone off of it. Our smartphones, and the apps that we've installed on them are the most distracting devices of our time. We are able to be with our loved ones and family however, we're texting, scrolling and interacting with our friends online. Sometimes, we are trying to capture our moments to display on a platform, and we miss the point when we should take it all in and enjoy it. Turn off your device so that you can concentrate. And, most importantly, be reminded of the goal of what you're doing.

* Meditation

The practice of meditation is about bringing yourself into presence. 10 minutes of practice every day will help to be more in the present. The practice could be as easy as spending a few minutes to pay attention to your breath or thoughts while staying present. It is possible to do it in the morning before beginning your day, or later at night when you wrap all of your activities or both.

* Practice

It doesn't need to be scheduled. If you've got just a few minutes it is possible to be present in your surroundings. Take a look around and observe tiny details you'd otherwise miss. Be sure to touch things and feel their feel Play some music and focus on listening to it. When you practice, concentrate on how these activities affect you.

Gratitude

When we practice Hygge We are thankful. We are grateful that we have the comfort of a fire and the warmth of our friends, the sweetness eating, the comfort of our blanket and the comfort of warm drink in your hands...the easy things.

When we feel happy with the little things, those which cost nothing We can then begin to observe and feel the abundance we have in our lives. If you're grateful for what you have, you feel content and are not thinking about the future looking around, hoping you could have something or another and getting anxious for lack of it. You are content with the present and are grateful for it, regardless of what is to be. According to research, a thankful one is more content, has a faster recovery from loss and stress and is more accepting and kind, which is the perfect recipe for happiness.

## Chapter 12: What to Make The Perfect Backyard Hygge Garden

It's time to transform your home to appear as a comfortable place to be in, even during the summer! Transforming your yard into an inviting space to recharge your batteries is the best method to give your own a gift which keeps on providing. Why should you buy points that will never bring you joy daily?

The key to creating a cozy life is spending the time needed to create a setting that allows you to relax and take in all that life has to provide.

Gorgeous illumination.

It is true that the way that stringing fairy lights around your home can transform it into a peaceful nook so why not beautify your outdoor space with some beautiful lights that instantly calm your soul?

See how stunning these lights are. You can feel the tension go away from your shoulders when you look at the lights.

Feathered friends.

I enjoy taking gardens scenic tours. The way others transform their homes to make everyone want to gather in their homes is what makes me happy.

The backyard that is etched in my head was planned out, so each part of it had a mark of individuality. The main thread that binds every component with the other was the owner's love for birds. They brought her joy.

Her yard was an area in which she could return the gift of all the happiness that they gave her, and delight them. They were happy I can tell you. The reason that this backyard is so prominent in my head is not only due to its aesthetics, but also as because of the number of birds were enjoying their own little oasis.

The birdbaths provided fresh water as well as protection from pests. She also had several bird feeders throughout the building to attract different species of birds. No pesticides were utilized in the garden , and there was very little grass in the yard -- mostly narrow pathways that were surrounded by yard beds everywhere.

Fruits that are a favorite.

What is your most loved fruit? Do you like lemons? How about some fruits like blueberries, raspberries, cranberries, tayberries , or strawberries? Do you get a giddy feeling from grapes when you think about them?

Create your own garden or tree to ensure you have an plenty of your favorite fruits all through the summer.

Themed garden.

Why would you want to have a garden at all and not have one with a theme that brings smiles to your face every time you look at it?

A few of the ideas you could consider are: fairy gardens or butterfly garden moonlight garden, a larger yard, pizza garden, cut-flower garden, fragrant garden, friend yard Shakespeare gardening, tea gardens are just some of the possibilities.

Fire to relax.

The idea of dividing a section of your backyard to create a fire pit is an perfect way to unwind in the evening , as and spend quality time with family and friends. It is possible to cook your favorite dinner dishes in it without heating your home with an oven. Aluminum foil-lined dishes are enjoyable and delicious, and they are simple to prepare.

Easy chair.

Find a comfortable lounge chair for star-gazing at night. There's no need to strain your neck in the chair when you could lie back and relax and enjoy the gorgeous night sky.

The ideal time to go stargazing is during August, as you can watch the Perseids meteor shower happens. The best days to view the Perseids meteor shower are August 11-13, 2018.

Alfresco dining.

There's no reason to remain inside eating your food during a hot summer day. As soon as the weather begins to heat up, you should plan to place all your food on a table outside and chairs.

Place your garden's blossoms in mason containers placed on the table to jazz things up. You should also check that your chairs are fitted with padding to ensure they're comfy for you on your own and with your family and friends. A key element of the hygge style of life is to enjoy in a relaxed and enjoyable time with your loved ones, and having an outdoor meal is a great way to do this.

Decorative touches.

Incorporating unique features to your garden such as concrete sculptures and mirrors, arbors, and iron garden gates will create an ambiance that is more relaxing. It is important to give your garden an "lived-in" appearance, so that you'll feel relaxed as soon as you walk out.

What is the best way to add some whimsy to your day?

Organic delight.

There's something about the scent of plants that boost our health. The great thing that pots of natural herbs in your backyard is that they don't take up lots of space. They not only smell amazing, but you also save some money because you don't have to buy these plants from the supermarket to prepare your meals.

It is also possible to preserve them in the winter months so you will be able to enjoy them throughout the all year.

Swing.

Isn't a single swing in the garden beautiful? Imagine how easy it would be to make a swing to your own heaven and then ask yourself why you've not set about setting the same thing before?

It's an easy way of giving that extra look back to the past to your everyday life.

The imaginative side.

Are you thinking of creating something distinctive to your backyard using your creativity? Mosaics are an excellent way to add beauty and elegance to any kind of backyard.

Mosaics can be used as accents for sculptures, walls or even stepping stones Gazebo.

A gazebo is a beautiful thing that is unmatched to me. Making sure your gazebo is in the right spot to enjoy the abundance your backyard has to offer is the best way to enjoy a day of your life.

Inspiring touches.

It's not likely that you want to create a complete fairy garden in your yard however, what about adding the smallest bit of imagination with the fairy pot or trees with an attached fairy door the trunk, or even some wooden tools or two? Why not expand the pots of four-leaf clover clovers to add your own luck?

Video games for yard.

The board games aren't the only way to challenge your family and friends to a bit of competition. Be sure to have a variety of games on the lawn like croquet or backyard bowling the ring toss and horseshoes or tennis for a bit of old-fashioned fun

Course winding.

There's something about winding courses in the yard that is distinctive. I switch the route to my front door one that winds in addition to going straight since it's meant to bring out the finest.

The Reasons Danes Get Danes

Are One Of The Happy Country

Denmark is known to be the "happiest nation in the globe." The reality is it is a semi-socialist paradise where medical treatment is free, and students receive a fee from the federal government to attend college, and the most popular pastime of all is curling up in front of a roaring flame with the glass of red wine, and an excellent guide. In 2017 Denmark was snubbed from the scratch on the World Joy Record through neighboring Norway however Danes have managed to rank at No. number one in happiness for 3 of the last five years.

Nordic countries have actually held the top spot in world happiness considering that the first Planet Joy Document came out in 2012, and this year's report isn't any different.

Five Nordic nations (Denmark, Finland, Iceland, Norway and Sweden) are rated among the top 10 on the basis of six essential criteria: freedom, generosity and wellness, as well as financial support, social assistance as well as a reliable administration. Although the GDP is greater than in the United States than all Nordic nations, Americans are still just the 14th most contented people on the planet.

Why are playing with LEGOs, eating pastry Danes winning the race for joy? We have reached out to Helen Russell, writer of The

Year of Living Danishly: Uncovering the Secrets of the World's Happiest Country to get information from a long-standing Londoner who relocated from London to Denmark just five years ago, and was also thrown off suddenly due to its tranquil, comfort-loving society. Here are the five reasons Russell cites for why Danes are more content than you.

According to research conducted, 79 percent Danes say they trust the majority of people. I'm not sure if that 79 percent of my current home," jokes Russell, who relocated out of Greater london to Denmark in 2013, when her husband received an assignment--where else?

Denmark's low population (far less than 6000) and its cultural consensus has something to do with it. However, the Danish perception of the world is broad, from neighbors who live next door to the authorities. Russell states that the majority of Danes don't secure their cars and car doors, or even the front doors.

Dependence isn't a innate Danish characteristic, Russell admits. Russell's book "The Year of Danish Living," Russell spoke with political analyst Peter Thisted Dinesen coming from Copenhagen College, that positioned that those from "low-trust" nations who have been educated in Denmark immediately deal with Danish trust levels.

It is the Danish Welfare Condition Functions

Danes have to pay for some of the highest tax rates in the worldforty-five percent for an average Danish annual income of $43,000, and 52 percent for individuals who exceed $67,000. In exchange for paying the majority of their earnings, each Dane is provided with free wellness care as well as free K-college education (pupils get paid $900 per month) and extremely subsidised youngster healthcare, as well as the chance to receive a charitable unemployment benefit. In research that show 9 out of 10 Danes say they are happy to pay for their tax burdens.

" The motivation behind the high degree of assistance for the state of wellbeing within Denmark is the awareness of how the wellbeing model transforms our wide spectrum right into health," develops Meik Wiking, primary executive officer of Denmark's Happiness Research Institute. "We do not have taxes.

If you lose your job in Denmark however, it's usually not an attractive offer. Due to a process known as"the "flexicurity method," companies in Denmark have even more discretion to dismiss employees due to federal programs that allow them to retrain employees and to better prepare them for the work market.

Denmark is also one of the most generous retirement programs in the world and is able to serve the over 65 population with a mixture of pension plans funded by the state and privately-owned, employee-funded pension programs. Also, if you're not constantly worried about the way you'll take care of your retirement it's likely that you'll experience less anxiety and more confident. That's right, you'll feel happier.

Danes are less productive and also Spend More time with their families

" The concept of balancing work-life" In Denmark isn't simply an Human Resources buzzword, it's an actual way of life. Danish employees are ranked in the lowest number of hours of any of the Organization for Economic Cooperation and Development (OECD) countries, with 1,412 hours a year. If Danes were employed for every week of the year, they would be only 27 hours per week. However, since the majority of Danish businesses use at minimum five weeks of paid vacation, Russell says that the true number is more like 33 hours a week. What is 33 hours in a week?

" As our family, we're mildly annoyed when my husband doesn't get home at

5:30 p.m.," states Russell who takes the maternity leave with twins who are 3 months old. "In London, we hardly ever saw each other."

In the area of parental leave for adults, Denmark once more has the most expansive policies in the world. The government requires all businesses to offer at least 52 weeks' parental leavefor mothers or dad. in addition, the state offers an amount of financial assistance that can be as long as 32 weeks.

For each and every days off Danish workers get, their the economy's performance doesn't appear to be impacted. According to OECD calculations of labor performance (GDP per hour of work), Denmark rates well above larger economies such as Germany, Japan and the United States. Russell credit ratings are a diverse workplace culture.

Denmark is "hygge headquarters. They also have a name for it,"hjemmehygge" (house Hygge). This might refer to the Danish love of beautiful design.

They also have the largest living spaces per person in Europe

" There's this idea that you put in the effort to finish the task and then you go home. Danes don't waste their time in the office by using Facebook," Russell claims. "You're further relying on your employer to perform great work, which is why you're in a position to work from home or set your personal schedule."

" Through all the work I've done in the area of joy research. This is the one thing I'm most confident about the most accurate predictor of whether or not is the social network we have.

Journalist Cathy Strongman, that moved from London to Copenhagen and who published on The Guardian: "Work later than 5:30. The work place is the morgue. Work on weekends and the Danes consider you insane. The thought is that families are able to relax and eat with one another at the close of the day throughout the day."

Denmark's People Don't Have Boasts

There's a law governing word-of mouth in Danish society that is known as Janteloven also known as "Jante's legislation,"based on a well-known mocking tale dating from the 1930s. The principle behind Janteloven can be described as "do not appear to be superior, smarter, or more wealthy than everyone other than you."

Janteloven has actually lost some of its hold in the cosmopolitan Copenhagen, Russell says, Janteloven is still largely inhabited by normal Danes (you might even say it's because being "typical" would be the aim).

Everyone is the same," claims Russell, noting that you won't find even the most wealthy Danes who drive fancy cars in lavish homes. "People are also dressed in casual attire and I've not noticed a connection for a while."

Not only are there fewer external indicators of victory or defeat, but failure in Denmark isn't an all-letters word, Russell states. Because Danes have such an extremely secure security net, there's not any financial risk for failure, which means that people are free to try new ideas. If they don't succeed it's not a big loss.

Danes Live Hygge-ly

To truly understand the factors that make Danes tick, and to understand why they're so happy and happy, you must understand the concept of hygge. Russell states that hygge is more than just crackling timber fires or pyjamas that fit your entire body it's anything that gives the soul to your core.

Russell says Russell claims that Danes are "bemused and even shocked" that hygge has become a popular self-help trend. An online search of Amazon provides over a dozen books on hygge that will reveal the

Danish way to be happy. This seems like a perfect book to quench that fire.

Drinks and food

"Sweets are Hyggelige. Cake is hyggeligt. Warm chocolate or coffee are both hyggeligt. Carrot sticks are but not many," Wiking states.

According to him, the high quality of confectionary, coffee, and even meat consumption in Denmark is directly related to hygge.

"Hygge refers to being nice to oneselfby giving yourself the opportunity to reward yourself in return for giving yourself, and one another to take a break from the pressures of a healthy lifestyle," he claims.

The Wiking's fellow Danes seem to be in agreement: the average Dane consumes 3 kilograms of bacon per year.

Christmas

Christmas is among the most cozy times during the whole year. "Even although it's possible to stay hygge-like throughout the year only once a year is the ultimate goal of an entire period," he says.

Xmas customs in Denmark aren't that different from those of the UK or United States, yet the different lies in the fact the fact that "a Danish Christmas will certainly always be planned, thought about and scrutinized in relation to the notion of Hygge."

There's also a term for it: the word julehygge (Christmas-hygge).

Lighting

From the famous lampshades to its staggeringly widespread lighting with candles, Denmark is a country who is obsessed with lighting. According to the Happiness Research Institute's research reveal that over 85% of Danes associate hygge with candles. 28 percent of Danes use candles every day.

Wiking refers to an American ambassador in Denmark that says candles create "a kind of happiness that is emotional as well as an feeling of emotional comfort."

# Conclusion

Denmark isn't just a place for its support of the winter cold It has been dubbed to be one of the more happy nations on the planet. Hygge might not be the best solution to all the challenges however If Denmark is any indication it's not going to cause any harm. Americans who live in warmer and cooler climates are experimenting with ways to take that perfect and comfortable look out of magazines and into real life. Although scan patterns for hygge were more prevalent in northern regions however, we did not find any limitations to the kind of urban communities or states that might attempt to adopt an progressively more agreeable and gentle approach.

Remember that hygge can be a lifestyle and you must invest in it and live it. Particularly it's not entangled with maintaining a perfect home. Don't also be stressed when things don't go exactly according to what you planned.

Hygge is the Danish concept of bringing happiness to everyday situations by creating the feeling of warmth and comfort is a concept that can be brought outside of the home and put into the workplace to ease stress and increase effectiveness.

www.ingramcontent.com/pod-product-compliance
Lightning Source LLC
Chambersburg PA
CBHW060329030426
42336CB00011B/1264